MW00588221

NIKSEN

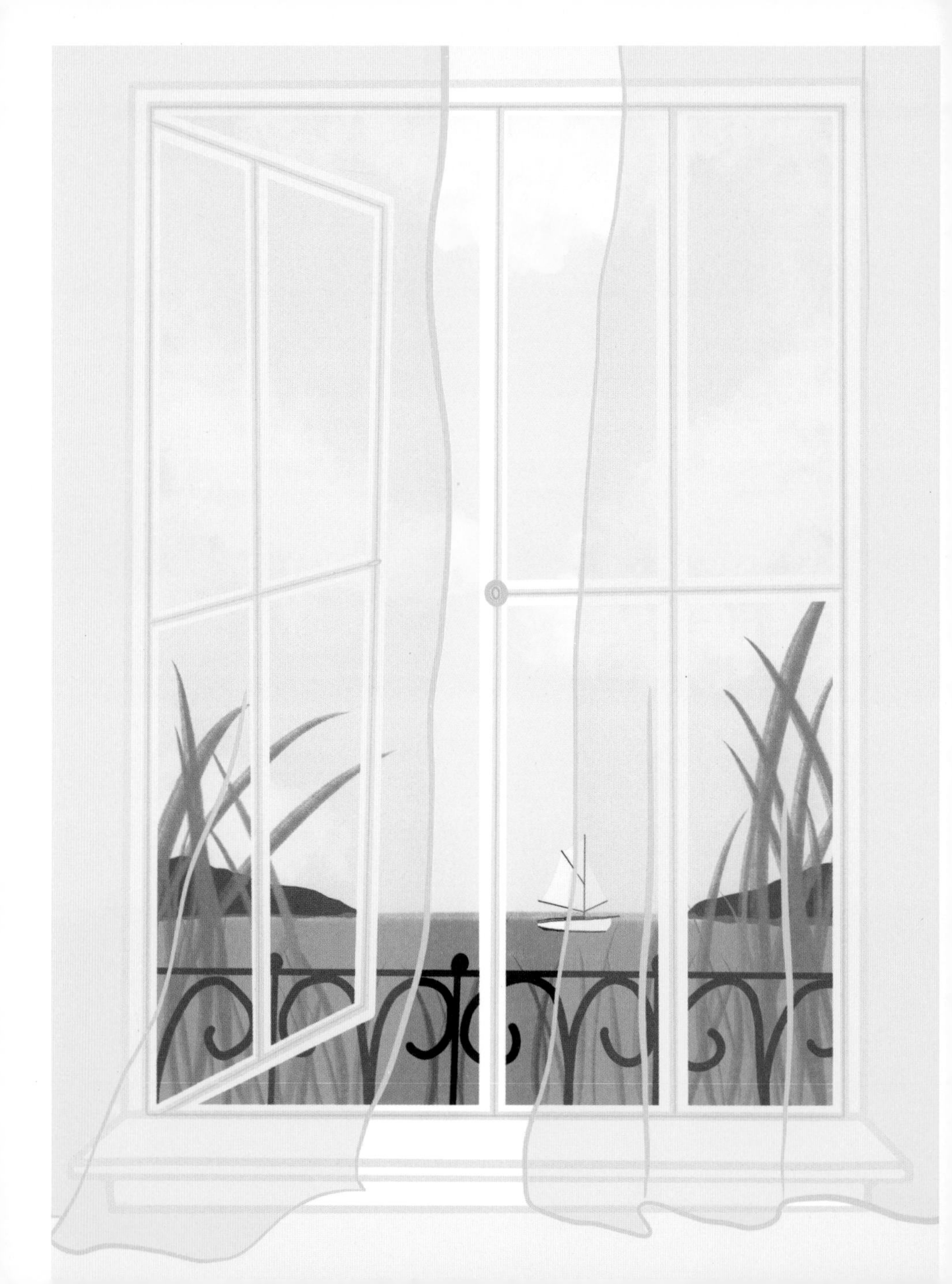

NIKSEN

The Dutch Art of Doing Nothing

Annette Lavrijsen

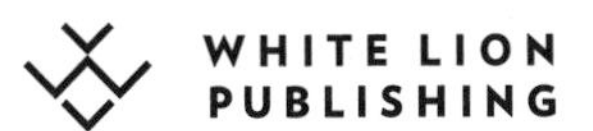

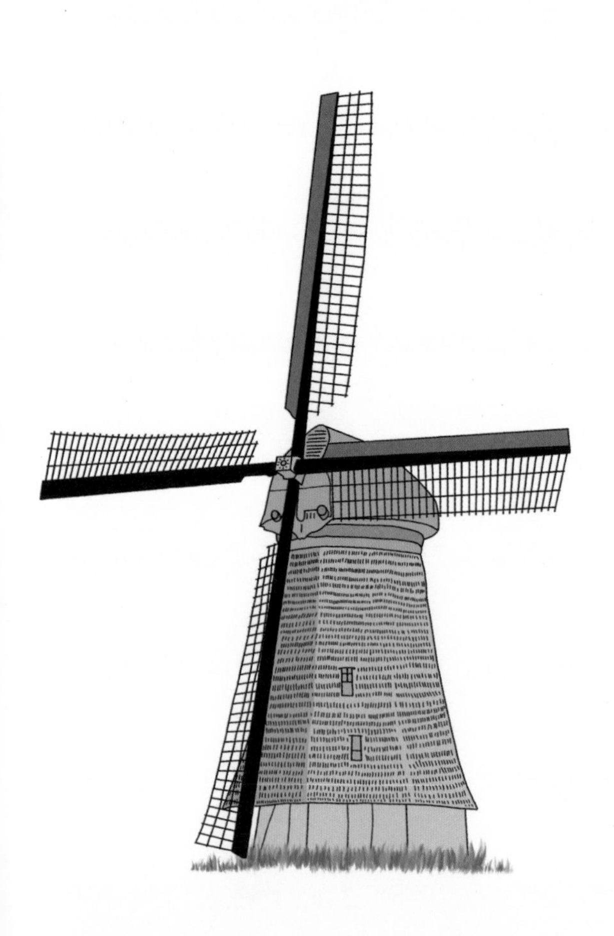

CONTENTS

INTRODUCTION

What is 'niksen' and why do you need it?

Imagine a world in which you stop trying to optimise every single moment, and instead spend your time on the things that truly matter. In short, you refuse to do everything in favour of, occasionally, doing nothing. This is niksen – the power of pause – the Netherlands' counterintuitive answer to almost any issue.

Lost? Stressed? Overwhelmed? Never reaching the end of that to-do list? Free yourself from external pressures and calm the chaos within by embracing niksen as a means of resisting our always-on culture. Use it to shed light on what you truly care about, and what you don't need to care so much about.

This sanity-saving book will show you the path to contentment. It is focused on helping you to prioritise yourself, to get you out of productive overdrive – no matter how busy you are – and to make every day better. It is designed to tame and eradicate all those pesky somethings that get in the way of nothing.

In Chapter 1, you will learn about niksen and the Dutch; how their amazing work–life balance is something you can have, too. Don't think you have time to do nothing? Chapters 2 and 3 explain why there's no excuses and how to reset your priorities. Chapters 4 and 5 show you how to master time management and carve out space for doing nothing in any environment. And in Chapters 6 and 7 we delve deeper into how a niksen state of mind and a healthy work–life balance lead to a happy, harmonious family life, and how to sustain all you have learnt.

I can't give you a how-to guide to doing nothing. It is intuitive and personal. It means putting your wellbeing first and, in turn, reaping the benefits. But getting there doesn't need to be hard. This book will help you develop a new attitude, through meditative exercises, simple tips and calming pursuits, to reach that all-important niksen lifestyle.

Treat this book as your first step to boosting your creativity, increasing your focus, improving your relationships and becoming a calmer and happier person, the Dutch way.

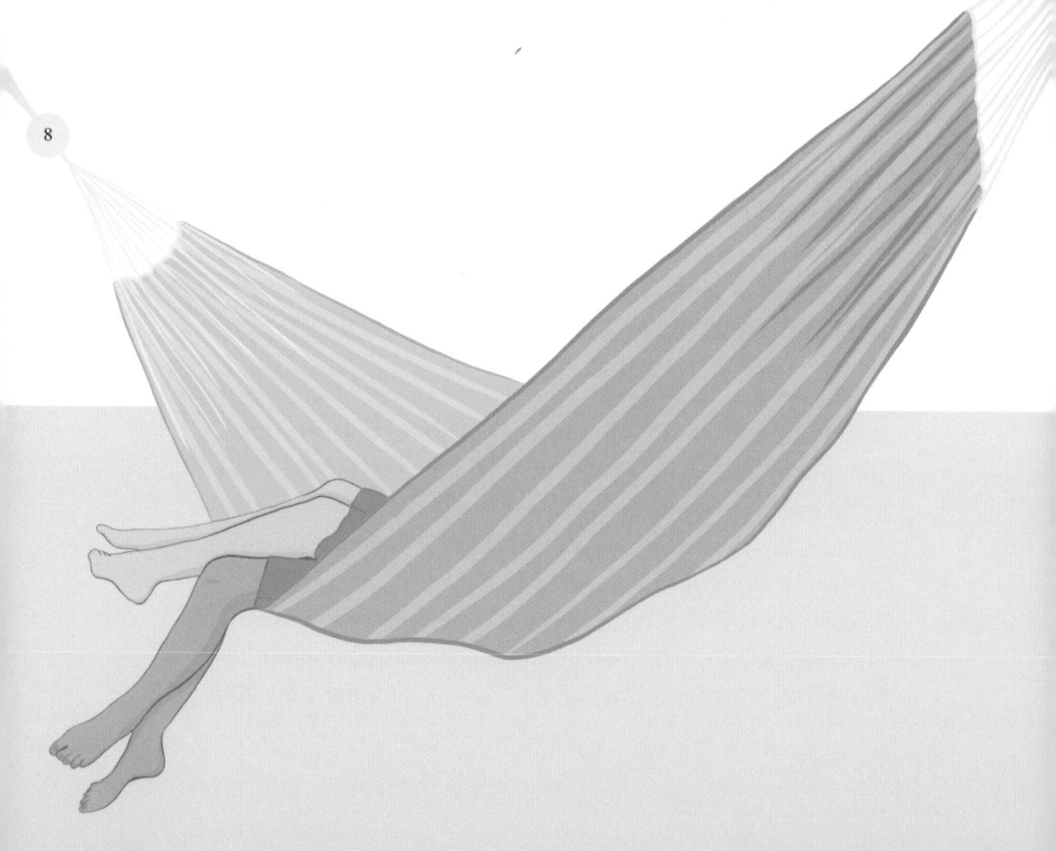

Fresh take on mindfulness

You may wonder if niksen is just another form of mindfulness. Well, not quite. You might have tried mindfulness before, taking a class or creating a sanctuary at home, complete with cushions, scented candles and a playlist full of mellow mantras. But how long did you last, really? You wouldn't be the first to give up long before enlightenment came into sight. Mastering mindfulness requires hard work and perseverance. Niksen, on the other hand, is far less complicated.

Niksen doesn't ask you to fold stiff limbs into the lotus position, or to practise until you can keep your mind from wandering (which for some may be forever). In fact, it doesn't require anything, except that you allow yourself a moment to do nothing, without a specific goal or purpose. And this is where it truly becomes interesting. Niksen can include any restorative pastime that takes your mind off your everyday worries, doesn't require any effort or headspace, and is useless in terms of generating profit, a fit body or social connections.

I know that, to the untrained eye, this may give the impression that you're just being lazy – antisocial even. But think about it: from improved creativity and self-confidence, to a higher self-awareness and reduced anxiety, doing nothing has the same restorative benefits as mindfulness – just with less effort. If you regularly take time out to allow your body and mind to rest and recharge, chances are you will eventually become a happier person, more relaxed parent, more effective worker, and a better friend.

Why you need niksen in your life

Niksen may not serve a direct purpose – it won't benefit your bank account, social network or figure – but a growing body of research is building the case for doing nothing in pursuit of greater productivity, creativity, health and happiness.

- **More energy**
  If you feel mentally depleted or exhausted, you can't be productive. By taking a timely break to do nothing, you can restore and recharge your body and mind.

- **Better health**
  Taking regular timeouts prevents you from running out of energy and focus, reducing the risk of burnout and other health problems.

- **Happier family**
  You will have more energy for your home life, allowing you to be more attentive to your family. Keep in mind that your kids will feel it if you are stressed and absent-minded.

- **A healthy brain**
  By keeping busy all the time, we lose our ability to sit still, reflect and be with our own thoughts. Research by the Dutch Donders Institute suggests being busy all the time can even alter the brain in a way that reduces our ability to think, focus and memorise things. A healthy brain needs downtime to restore the damage done.

- **Greater efficiency**
  Having developed your power to focus, you'll get tasks done much more efficiently.

- **Enhanced self-awareness**
  Minimalise and declutter your calendar by being selective: don't waste your time and energy on tasks that have no value. You will also gain more insight into the things that are (really) important to you.

- **The possibility of an epiphany**
  When we retreat our minds from our daily routines, we are able to look at problems, questions and issues with more distance and clarity. In turn, we become more resourceful, and may come up with creative ideas and solutions.

- **More time for planning long-term goals**
  Research published in the journal *Consciousness and Cognition* in 2012 reports that when we allow our minds to wander, we think about the future and long-term goals fourteen times more often than when we force ourselves to focus. Niksen can therefore result in goal-setting.

- **Better sleep**
  If we are plugged in at all times, immediately responding to every email and text, always alert, it becomes impossible to relax and quiet our minds to fall asleep. By building in more breaks during the day, you can reduce your stress levels and improve your sleep quality.

1

THE HAPPY DUTCH

Measuring roughly 41,500 km^2 (16,023 mi^2), the Netherlands is one of Europe's smallest countries. It is also continuously ranked as one of the happiest nations in the world. So what are they getting so right?

The Dutch and Niksen

Relatively small income disparities, a high standard of living and a stable political climate in which people are free to make their own life choices undoubtedly all play a major role in keeping this nation chirpy. Some, however, attribute the fact that the Dutch are happier than most other countries to their balanced approach to work, leisure and parenting. And they may be on to something. In 2019, the Better Life Index ranked the Netherlands as the country with the best work–life balance in the OECD[1], leaving even the Scandinavian strongholds behind.

	Dutch	**OECD**
% Employees working 50+ hours	0.4	11
	Dutch	**EU**
Average weekly work hours	29.3	36.2
% Female part-time workers	73.8	32.3
% Male part-time workers	27.4	9.8

Source: stats.oecd.org

You can only stay healthy, creative and happy if you also allot time to slowing down, taking a break and, most importantly, taking care of yourself. This is where niksen comes in.

1 *Organisation for Economic Co-operation and Development: www.oecd.org/countries*

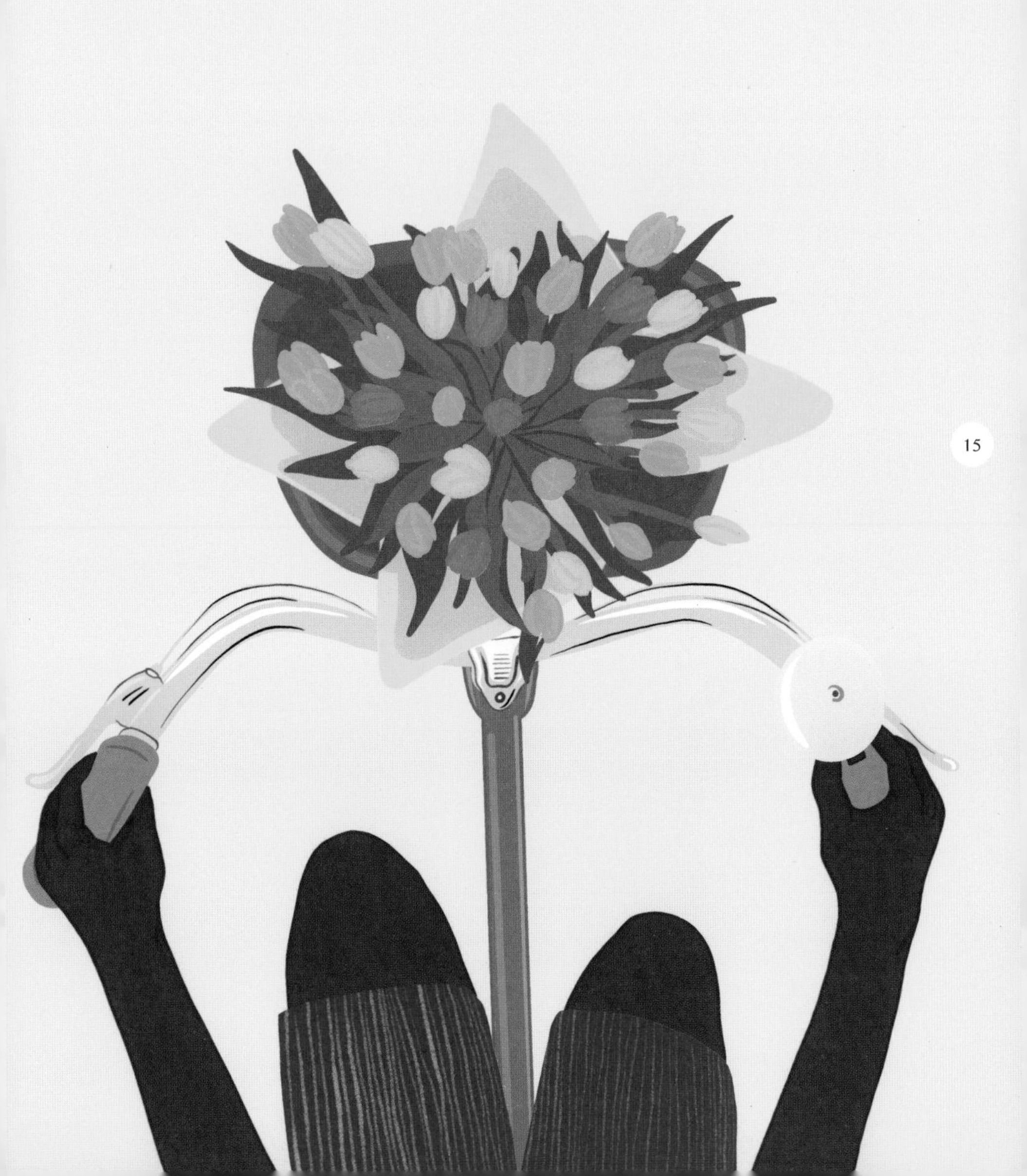

A Nation of Niksers?

For the Dutch, the verb *niksen* has long-held negative connotations. Whoever was caught niksing – as in, doing nothing useful – was accused of being lazy, useless and good for nothing (see page 18). Blame it on the old Calvinist virtues of hard work, capital generation and frugality, which Dutch society was once built on, and which over the years have become known as typical Dutch traits. From childhood, Dutch people learn to work hard and be productive. Even in their free time, many feel they should make themselves useful – by doing chores around the house, taking a course, or by volunteering.[2]

That niksen is currently being reinterpreted as a positive practice undoubtedly has to do with the way our lives have changed. The world today is faster, noisier, more connected and more fragmented than ever. It feels impossible to switch off, to disconnect and stop, and it would be naive to assume that the Dutch have remained blissfully unaffected by the stressors of modern life. It makes those moments of nothingness even more valuable and necessary.

---

2 *In the 2019 World Happiness Report, 35.6 per cent of the Dutch population claimed to have volunteered in the past month.*

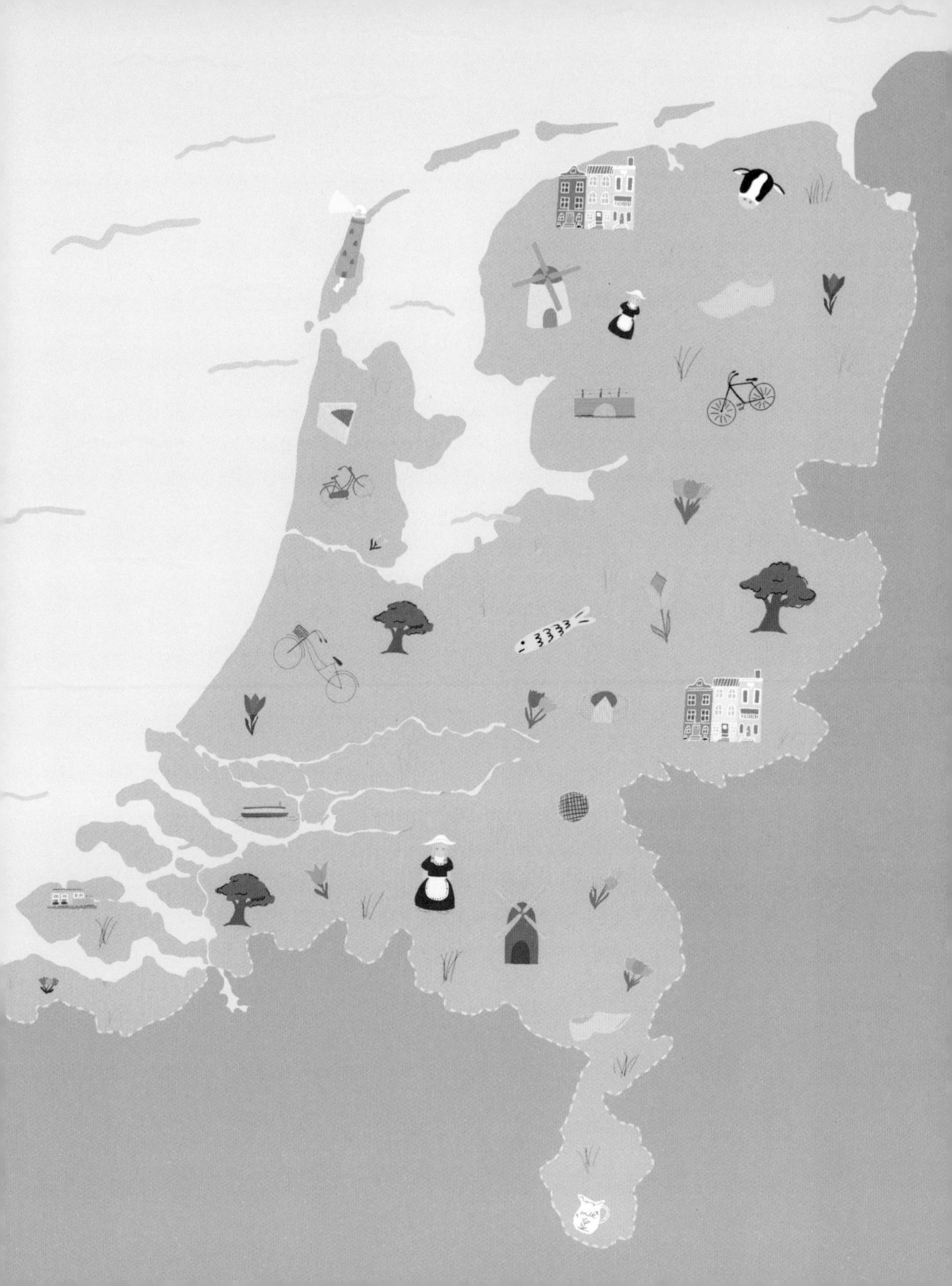

What's in a Name

The *Van Dale* (the leading dictionary of the Dutch language) simply says 'doing nothing' under the heading *niksen*. While the indefinite pronoun *niks* was already commonly used in the eighteenth century, *niksen* seems to be a relatively new word that has evolved from colloquial usage in the 1920s.

Someone who is doing nothing is sometimes called a *niksnut*, by which one means (as a joke or seriously) that this person is good for nothing. But the word is also now resurging with positive connotations – the Dutch are embracing a lifestyle where sometimes wasting time does not automatically get dismissed as wasteful.

Niksen can be used in combination with: *zitten (te) niksen* (most common), *staan (te) niksen* or *lopen (te) niksen*, meaning *niksen* while you're sitting, standing or walking respectively. The ultimate is of course *liggen (te) niksen*, meaning *niksen* while lying down on a bed, on a sofa, on the grass, etc.

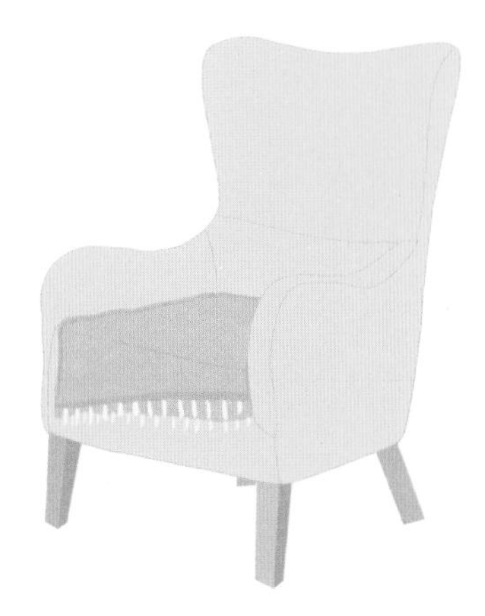

I remember...

As a child, whenever I was lying on the sofa after school, my parents would tell me off and find me a chore to do. Niksen was a useless pastime, my parents said, something for a lazy Sunday and the Christmas holidays. I rebelled. Whenever I saw an opportunity, I would retreat to the woods behind our house. Unhindered by time, I would plough through the thick layer of leaves on the ground, climb up and sit in a tree, or lay flat on my back to watch the dragonflies, birds and clouds float by, while my mind meandered.

Now well into my thirties, I still feel the pressure to fill my free time with purposeful, goal-oriented activities. Even leisure pursuits require an investment of attention and energy. But I wouldn't be able to keep all these balls in the air if I didn't carve out time too for those moments of niksen my parents scolded me for, in which I can enjoy my own company and be alone with my thoughts.

Getting Started

Before you begin, here's what you need to know about what, where, how and when to practise niksen.

What

Niksen literally means 'to do nothing' – nothing more, nothing less. It's about those brief moments in life when we press pause and retreat from our everyday work and social events, allowing ourselves to be idle, unhindered by feelings of guilt or thoughts about all the things we should be doing. As it does not require any special skills, it is accessible for everyone. Niksen usually doesn't involve sleeping – which is a different verb (*slapen*), for good reason – but one thing can obviously lead to another, and if you can't resist closing your eyes, go ahead.

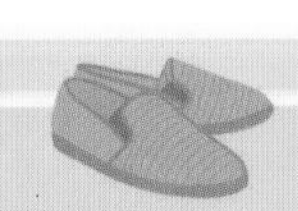

Having doubts about allowing all this nothingness into your life? On pages 30–41 you'll find a few myth-busting truths about niksen, to put your mind at rest.

Why Binge-watching is Not the Best Sort of Niksen

Binge-watching a whole season of your favourite show in one evening might seem like niksen – but it can actually lead to higher levels of stress, anxiety and depression. When we binge-watch, our brain produces dopamine, the same chemical that's associated with addiction. This explains why we often feel low after the final episode of a series. Try to limit your streaming time and decide beforehand how many episodes you're allowed to watch. Set your alarm as a 'wake-up call'.

Where

Retreat to a peaceful place where you feel calm and at ease, such as a bench in the corner of your garden, a nearby park or forest, a spa or a quiet space in the office or house (see page 83). If you are at home, put on some music, fill up the bathtub or retreat to the sofa and create a *gezellige* atmosphere (see overleaf). If you don't have an actual physical place to go to, you can daydream and mentally travel to your happy place.

A Companiable Atmosphere

Gezelligheid **is the Dutch equivalent of** ***hygge*****, the Danish concept of creating a cosy, warm atmosphere that promotes wellbeing. There is a subtle difference, however: while hygge reveres the closed-off cosiness of one's own home,** ***gezelligheid*** **(originating from the word** ***gezel*****, meaning 'companion') evokes a sense of sociability. It can be used to describe a fun get-together with friends, a sociable person or – in the context of niksen – a room with an inviting ambience.**

EXERCISE

BRING IN SOME GEZELLIGHEID

We usually put effort into creating a convivial atmosphere when we have visitors, so why wouldn't you do the same when you are alone?

Dim the lights, light a few candles and put your favourite playlist on to set the mood for niksen and for the better enjoyment of your own company.

How

Finding it difficult to relax without any external stimulation? Try doing one thing purely for the sake of it. This feeling of stepping out of oneself and out of time holds the promise of arrival in a state of flow, far away from your day-to-day concerns.

- An easy walk in nature, without a phone or watch, can help you ease into downtime (see page 88).

- Semi-automatic activities turn our hands and attention to something other than work (see page 129).

When

Niksen's true potential lies in the small pauses of everyday life. Don't put too much pressure on yourself to relax by waiting until the weekend or your summer holiday, knowing that this is your only opportunity. The trick is little and often. It is essential to make niksen part of your day-to-day routine, whether at work (see page 84) or within the confines of your home (see page 78).

Carve out time in your daily schedule: start by taking a timeout of five minutes (yes, also from your devices), gradually building it up to 30 minutes (see page 69), an hour or even a complete afternoon. Dedicate this time to you and you alone, keeping in mind that it is okay to sometimes do nothing. It really is.

EXERCISE

ARE YOU NIKSING?

If you're not sure that what you're doing is niksen, then ask yourself three questions:

Am I doing something useful or productive?

Am I doing this to impress my boss or business relations?

Will this directly benefit my social connections?

If you can answer **no to one of these questions**, you may be niksing. To be certain, have a look at the following statements:

This is costing me zero physical effort or headspace, and afterwards I feel calmer and more relaxed.

I have unplugged fully, unhindered by thoughts of all the (more useful) things I should be doing instead.

If anyone saw me now, they would think I am just being lazy – and I don't care.

If **all three statements are true**, it is very likely that you are niksing.

If not, think of the moments that do tick all the boxes. Can't think of any? You've opened the right book.

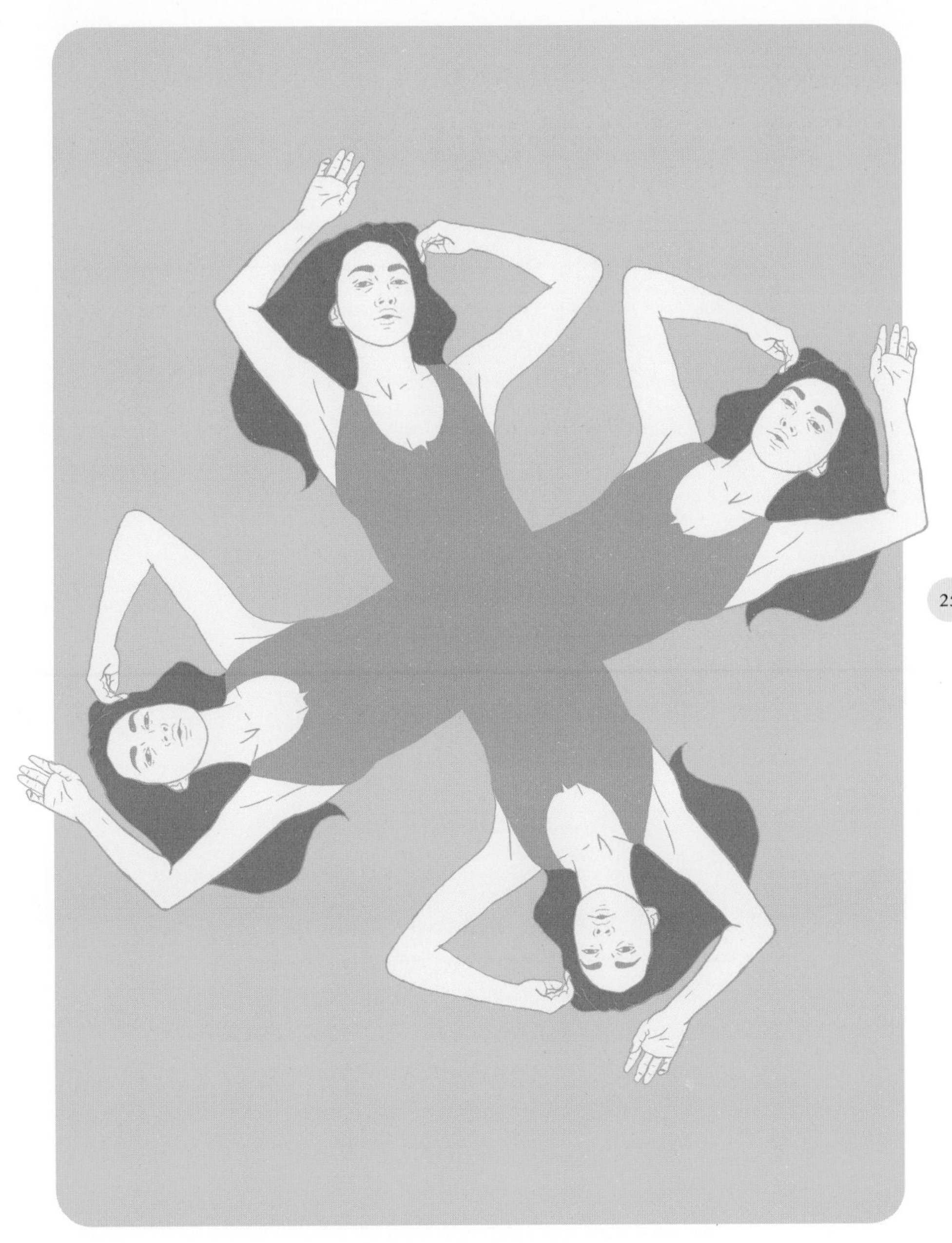

A MANIFESTO OF NIKSEN

1

I will make doing nothing a priority,
because I know it will help me become more productive, more creative, and an overall healthier and more content person.

2

I will allow myself to do nothing,
even if that means I'm being unproductive or antisocial in that moment. And I will ignore anyone – friend, colleague or inner critic – who says that doing nothing is synonymous with being lazy, counterproductive or selfish.

3

I will carve out time to do nothing every day,
by setting healthy boundaries that create space in my calendar and in my mind, and through improved time management.

4

I will make these moments of nothingness an integral part of my professional and private life,
and invite niksen's life-changing potential into my life.

5

I will make doing nothing a habit for life,
dedicating time to passive and active relaxation and non-goal-oriented activities which allow my mind to unwind and wander.

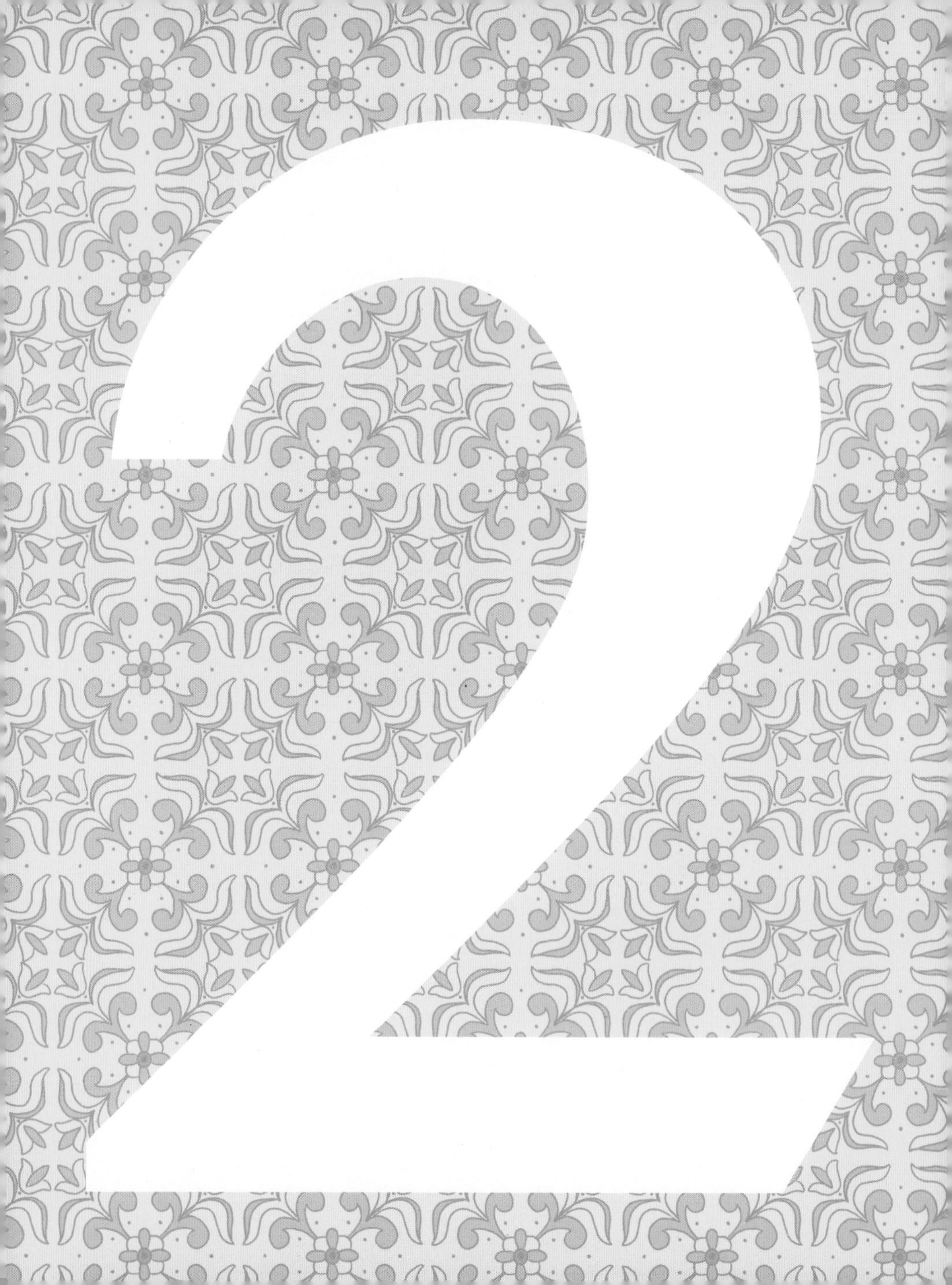
2

DARE TO BE IDLE

Doing nothing may seem easy at first, but when you actually start making it part of your everyday routine, things can get complicated. What is keeping us from claiming these timeouts to rest and recharge? Once you understand why it's so difficult for you to simply do nothing, you can start using the tools in this guide to slowly transition into a more balanced person who makes the most of life by pressing pause.

Myth Busting

I'm too busy at work . . . I can't unplug . . . I can't disappoint my friends . . . I can't . . . The list of excuses we come up with seems endless. Why don't we just allow ourselves to indulge in some nothingness every now and then, especially when those moments of self-care will help us better achieve our goals in the long run? Let's have a closer look at the underlying beliefs that keep us from doing nothing.

Practise Dutch Generosity

Gunnen is the selfless act of wishing another person a positive experience or success without expecting anything in return – particularly on occasions when it is earned ('_Het is je van harte gegund_', meaning 'I hope you'll enjoy it, you've earned it'), and even if it denies you the same experience. **See page 34 for how to practise this.**

It should be something that lifts your mood, so if it creates high levels of stress instead, then you need to rethink the scale of the gesture. Be generous on your own terms and, most importantly, be generous to yourself as well. A common Dutch expression used to describe stressed people as '_Zich geen rust gunnen_' ('Not letting oneself pause and rest'). You too deserve the generosity you may only reserve for those around you. Treat your mind by giving yourself a break.

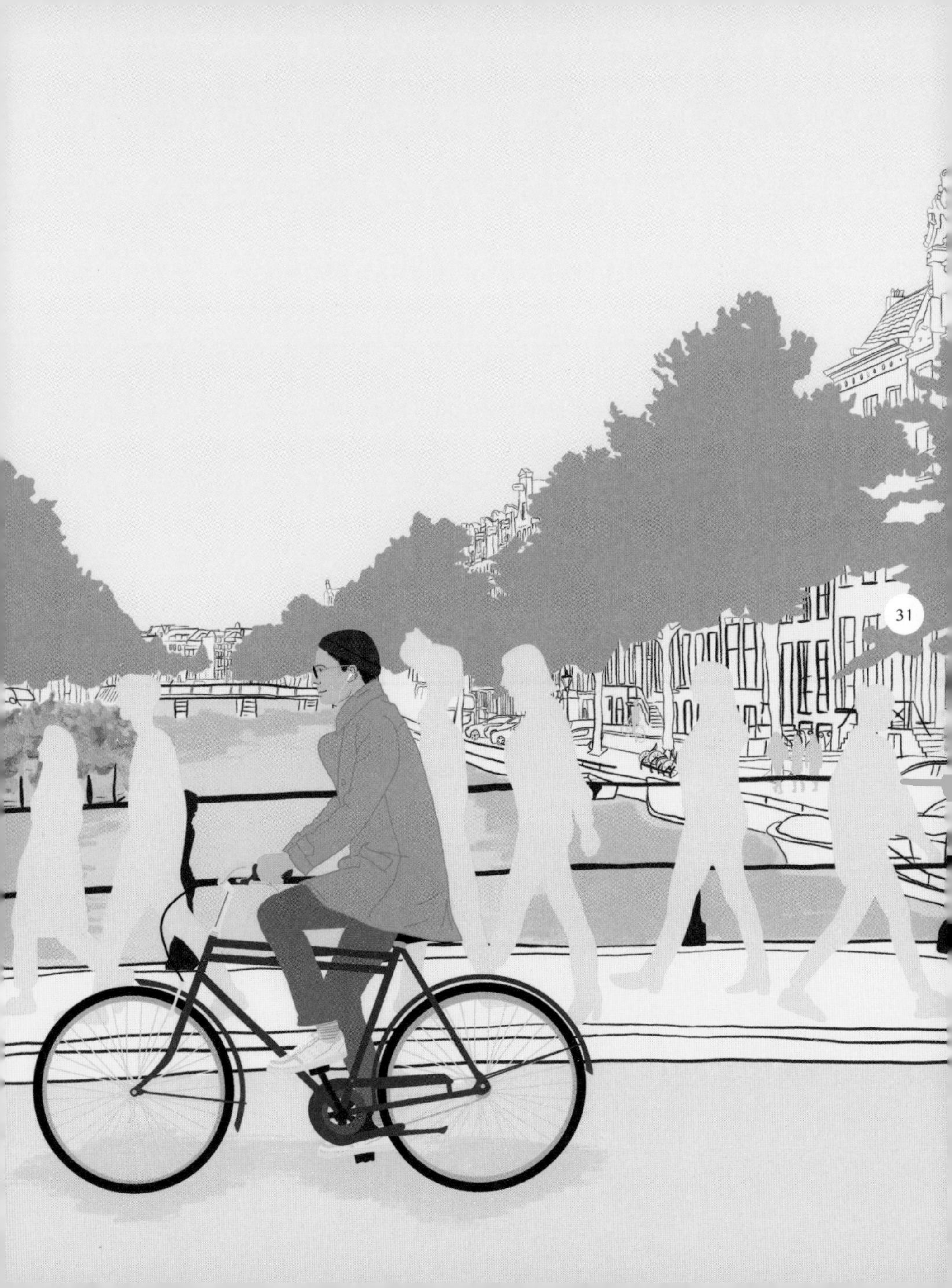

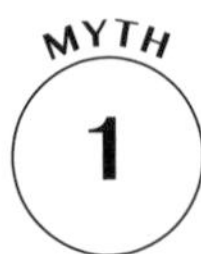

I'm too busy to do nothing

Being busy has become synonymous with being successful. We have been raised with the belief that we can climb the social ladder or turn any passion into a commercial success, if only we work hard enough.

The little voice in your head that says you should put the brakes on is muted with a simple 'No can do, I'm too busy.' Do you honestly believe you don't have the time to add a few pauses to your day? What you probably mean is that you don't want to invest time in just doing nothing, because you're afraid it might harm your productivity. After all, time is a luxury, and you better spend it wisely.

But what if the best use of your time is to start putting yourself first? If you keep accepting new projects and invitations at the expense of rest and recovery time, it will have a negative impact on your health in the long term. Of course, it requires courage to push the brake; it means you have to admit to yourself and to others that you're not a superhero and that you can't do everything. But which activities and tasks should you take out of your schedule in favour of doing nothing, when everything seems equally important? The following exercise can help.

EXERCISE

ARE YOU SPENDING TIME ON THE RIGHT THINGS?

Suppose your week had eight days instead of seven.

Which activities – leisure or professional – would you add to the week?
What new plans would you start working on?

Your answers will tell you something about the things that are a priority for you, but that you don't have time for right now.

Now suppose there are only six days in the week.

This means your time has suddenly become even more valuable.

Which activities would you give priority to?
And to which areas of your life would you give less time?

Ask yourself the above questions now and again, to find out whether you're spending your time on the things that matter most, and whether you're spending enough time on doing nothing.

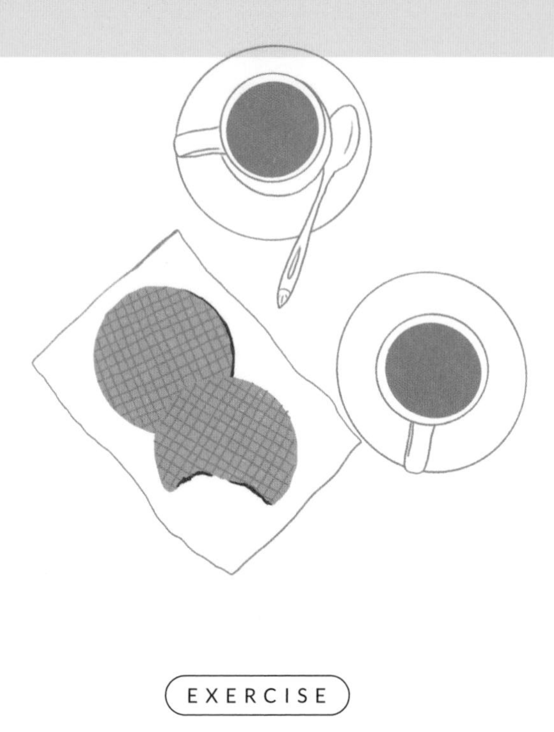

EXERCISE

PAY IT FORWARD

Psychologists have found that when we experience the kindness of another person, it is more likely that we are then kinder towards others, thus creating a domino effect. And the act of generosity, and the gratitude we receive in return, is good for our own mood, too. It helps us to get out of our own head for a bit. But we should know our limits and remember that we are no less important than others.

The following pointers should help you find the right balance:

①

Start by raising your awareness and notice the
many acts of generosity by others.

②

Look for opportunities to be generous every day,
but on your terms: don't sell those concert tickets – give them
to a friend; pass that cool project on to your co-worker
to create more space in your schedule.

③

Don't offer anything more than what is within your means.
If a favour endangers your personal downtime,
you're entitled to say no.

④

If someone is generous to you and offers help, appreciate it.
Instead of brushing it off or saying 'you didn't have to do that', simply
say 'thank you' and give them a smile.

Do this every day for at least a week and count the number of smiles it brings you.

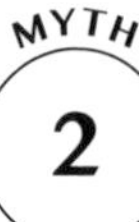

Nothingness is laziness

How often do you find yourself multitasking: commute, emails, texts, calls, instant messaging, meetings, work, home . . . When are you not plugged in? And are you actually getting anything meaningful done? The world today is faster, more connected and more frenzied than ever. Doing nothing seems inexcusable, a sin. We seem to have forgotten how to sit still with our own thoughts.

It's not that we don't yearn for nothingness: mindfulness retreats and sabbaticals have never been so popular. And yes, these clean breaks are certainly beneficial – we feel re-energised and motivated to pursue our goals – but how long do these effects last?

Nothingness should not be treated as a one-off indulgence, but thought of as a long-term solution. It acts as the tonic to the madness, calming the soul and promising clarity. It feeds insight and productivity, rather than busyness. It forces you to stop, and helps you to start. We need our daily dose of pause. We need to start saying no. And we need to remember that time is not money; time is our own.

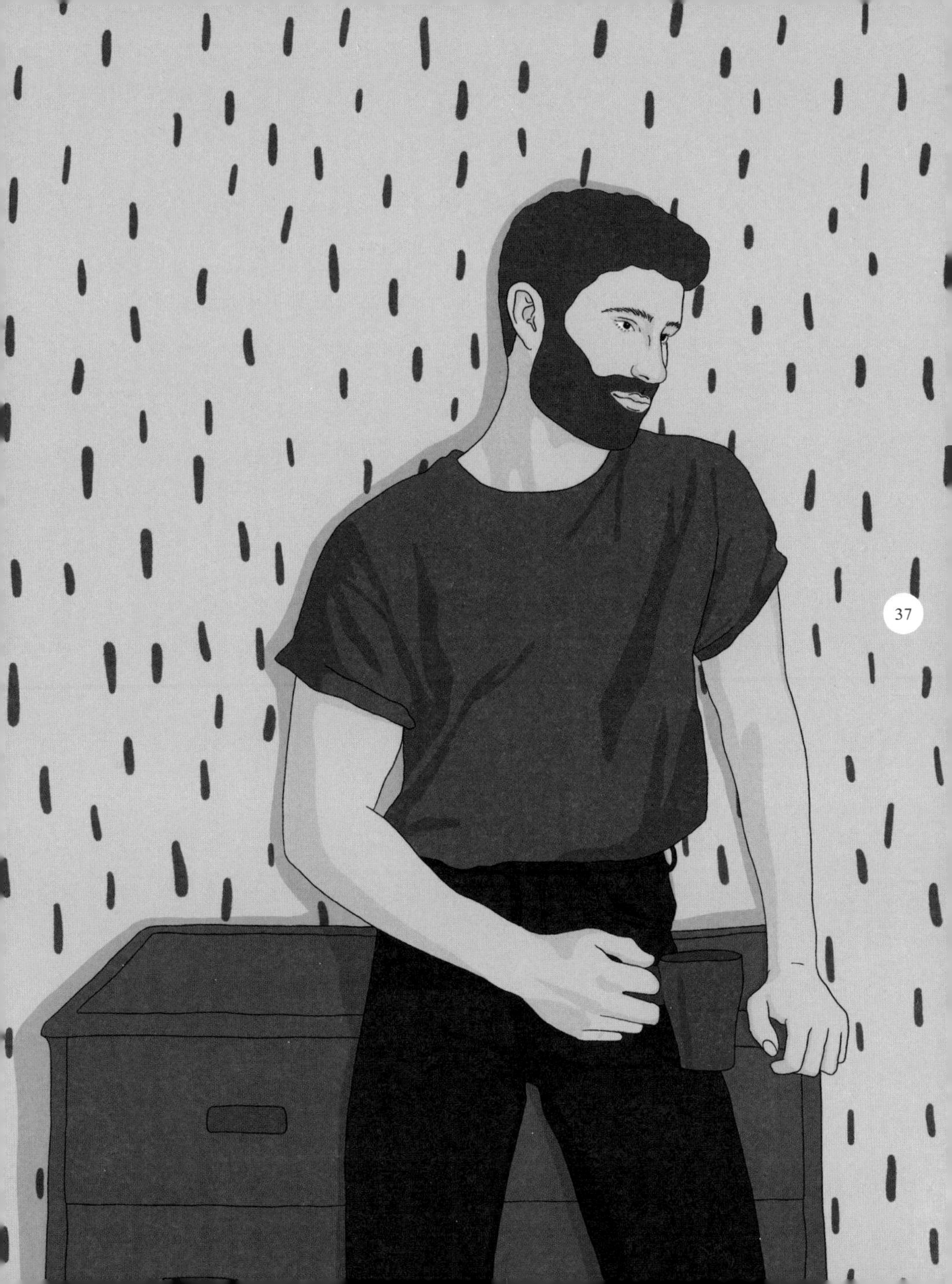

EXERCISE

NO MORE EXCUSES

I need to be available twenty-four seven . . . I have too many responsibilities to be lazy . . . My boss will fire me . . . If you find it difficult to keep the excuses from piling up, the following Viking-style ritual may help you bid them farewell. For this ritual you will need a candle, a fireproof bowl, a box of matches, a stick of palo santo ('holy wood') and a piece of paper and pen.

STEP ① Place the candle in the fireproof bowl and light it. Then light the palo santo stick and wave its scented smoke into the room. It is said that the woody scent helps to clean up negative energies and has an uplifting effect on mood.

STEP ② Write down all your excuses for why you can't make time to do nothing.

STEP ③ Fold the paper and hold your excuses in both hands while you close your eyes.

STEP ④ Say your goodbyes to your excuses, and tell them to go ruin another party. Then hold the paper with all your excuses on it in the candle flame and burn it to ashes.

STEP ⑤ Light the palo santo stick again and imagine how its smoke cleans up the energy created by the burned excuses, leaving you feeling lighter and more positive.

This may all feel a bit silly, but what you are doing with this symbolic ritual is telling yourself that these excuses are no longer yours to claim. Repeat the ritual whenever you feel it's needed.

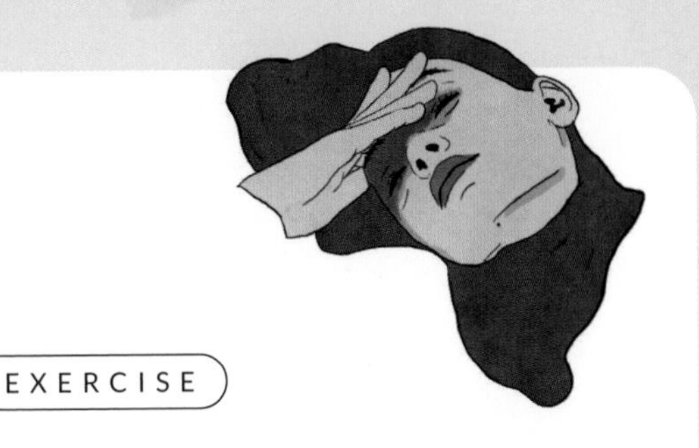

EXERCISE

SORRY NOT SORRY

Whenever we are not being productive, we feel guilty:

I have done the wrong thing, because all I did this morning was have breakfast, check Instagram and stare out of the window.

I failed to do the right thing, because I didn't finish the report I was due to send in this week.

It's easy to beat yourself up, even though the world hasn't ended. And taking a break to do nothing is another instance where no crime has been committed. So rewrite the narrative. Think of reasons why you were doing nothing that won't make you feel guilty.

I have done nothing wrong, because I listened to my body which was craving some time off.

I needed to see things at a distance, and stopping helped me to have clarity.

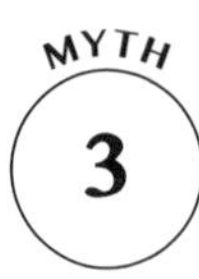

It's bad to take time out because people need me

Ask yourself: why do you care so much about what other people think of you? Are you afraid they will be disappointed in you or think you're a bad and selfish person?

Most of us have been raised with the idea that we should care for others, that it would be self-centred and arrogant to put our own needs first. However, if you continuously sacrifice your free time in favour of other people, you're burning the candle at both ends until you have nothing left to give.

If you want to feel indispensable and needed, this is your wake-up call. Remember the emergency instructions in the plane? You can only help others if you put your oxygen mask on first. You are no use to anyone if your energy is depleted because you have given every last bit of it away. Yes, support others, but nurture yourself first. Stop wasting your energy through this need to feel needed, and start investing more time in the most valuable person in your life: yourself.

EXERCISE

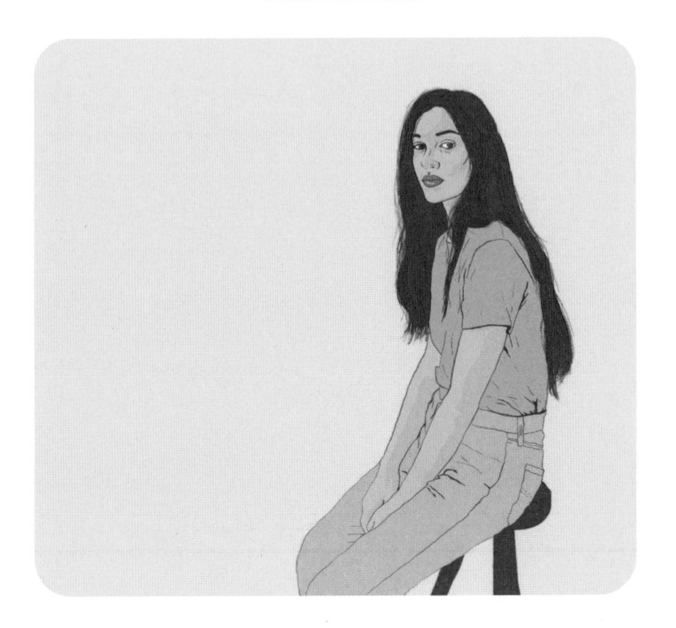

THINK BACK...

. . . to the last time you said yes to something you didn't want to do because you found it difficult to say no.

Why was saying no so hard? Be honest with yourself.

What could you have done differently, in hindsight?

What would have been the consequences if you had said no?

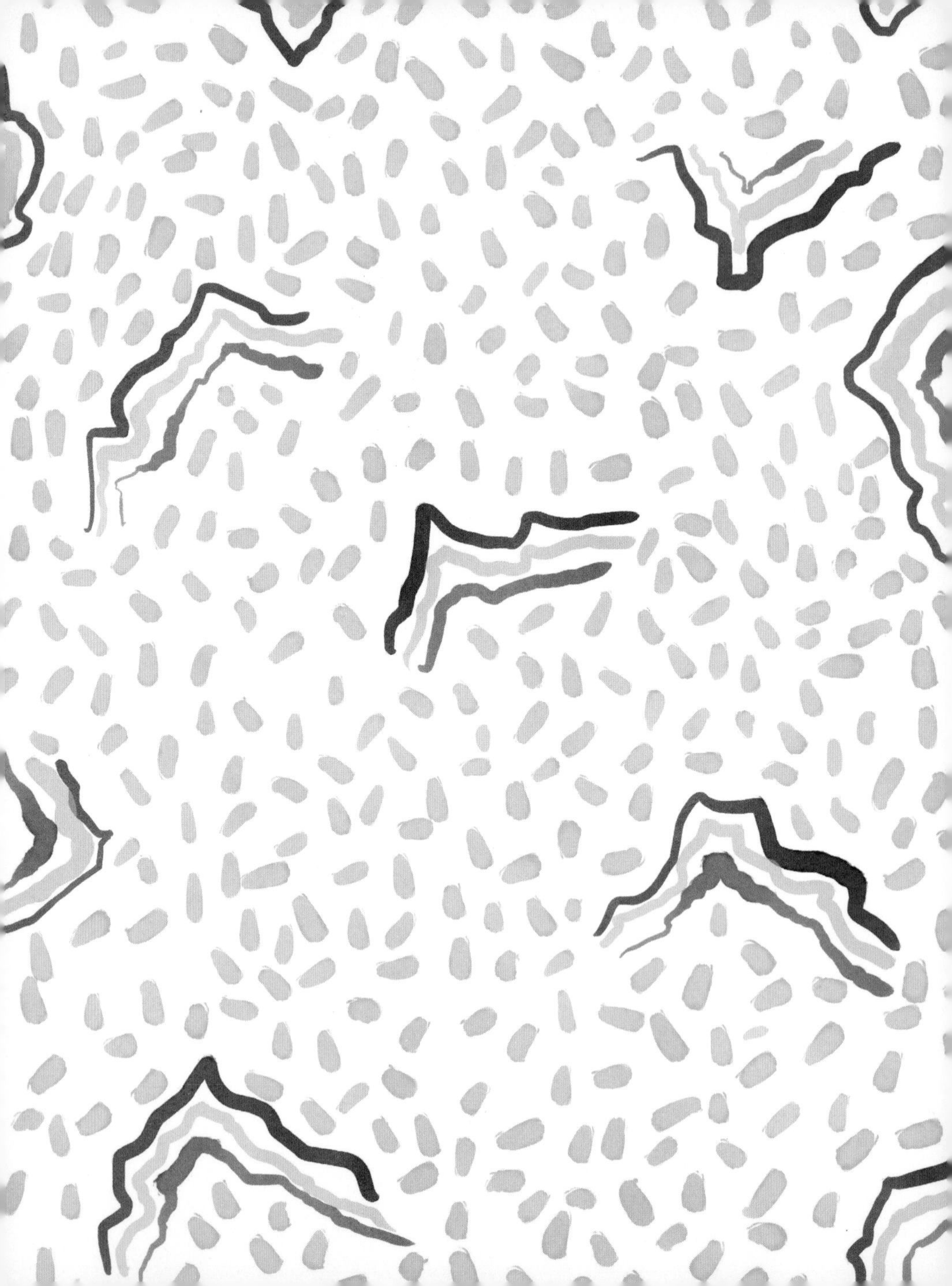

Positive Affirmations

An affirmation is simply a statement – thought, spoken aloud or written down – which can act as a powerful tool in encouraging you to do something, including nothing. We affirm things all day long, when talking to others and in our own head, but unfortunately many of us are affirming negative thoughts that do not serve us. When it comes to doing nothing, we sabotage ourselves with affirmations like:

Doing nothing won't help me advance my career . . .
I am a lazy pig . . . Passivity is bad . . .

If you repeat these affirmations often enough, you will start to believe them. So change the dialogue. Use positive affirmations to build your self-esteem and encourage daily timeouts:

I listen to my body when it's telling me it's tired . . .
If I rest now I can be more productive later . . .
It's okay to do nothing . . .

A Dutch person would probably say it requires *moed* to block that negative, doubting voice at the back of your mind that pushes against these positive phrases. *Moed* is the inner courage to follow your gut feeling, despite what others may say, or think, or expect from you. It's a positive trait and should not be mistaken for bravado or boldness, which is intended to impress or intimidate others – this is about you, not them. By repeating positive affirmations every day, you will train your brain to be more *moedig*.

EXERCISE

LET GO OF THE PAST

Many people's minds are sponges for mistakes made, opportunities missed and grudges or grievances held. All these feelings and memories are like the sandbags hanging from a zeppelin, slowing it down and preventing it from flying and discovering new lands. Take time to identify these sandbags and cut loose anything that doesn't serve you anymore. Off with it! You live in the now, and this clutter is only wasting your time and energy.

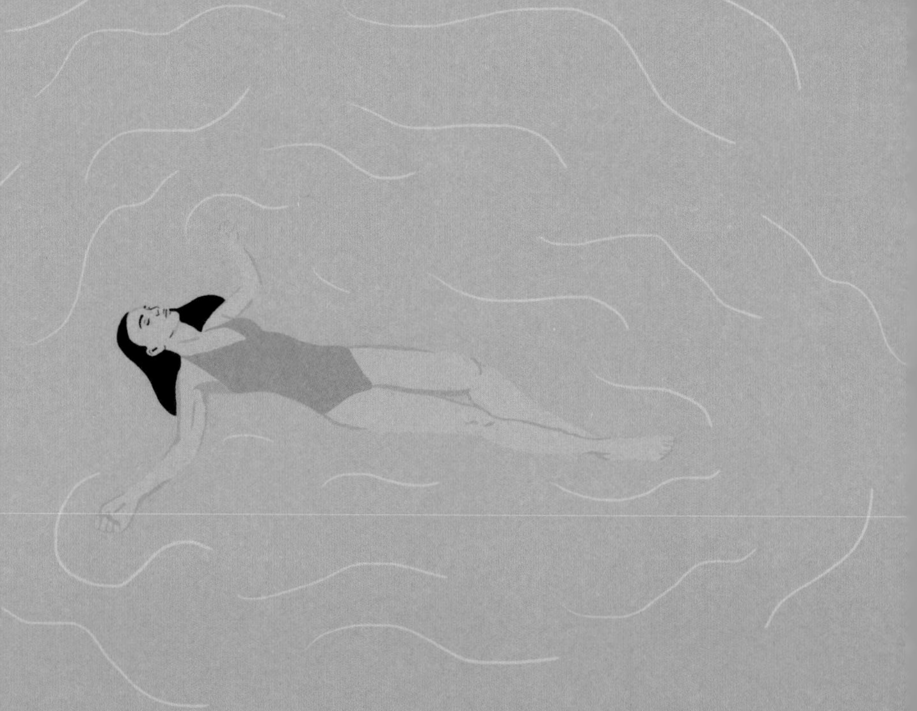

EXERCISE

IT'S OKAY

In your notebook or journal, write down the phrase 'It's okay to do nothing', and read it out loud. Write the same phrase again, read it out loud again, and repeat as often as needed, until you start believing it (or until you can't feel your fingers anymore).

Want to use your own affirmation? Go ahead. You can find inspiration in the list below. Just make sure it's something you want deeply, and keep it positive and authentic.

It's okay to put my best interests first and to...

- not answer a call.
- say no to something I don't want to do.
- stay home on a Saturday night.
- take the afternoon off.
- take a day off.
- cancel a commitment.
- change my mind.
- do nothing.

RESET YOUR PRIORITIES

Niksen creates balance. You have to make time for it and in doing so, you need to take a long hard look at your schedule. Timeouts can actually make us think more clearly and be more productive. Learn to enjoy more of your day by taking a breath and refocusing your energy to best tackle your tasks, and find more time for the things you love. And remember that before you can start niksing, you need to get your priorities sorted.

Act Normal, Already

If there's one saying that defines the Dutch national character, it must be '*Doe normaal, dan doe je al gek genoeg*', which roughly translates as 'Just act normal, that's crazy enough already'. This expression is deeply embedded in Dutch culture and reflects the socio-cultural norm to not show off or act pretentious, not brag about how much money you make, and not display any extravagant, attention-seeking behaviour. Ambitious overachievers who slave away their life are pitied with a '*Niet normaal*' ('Not normal'), even if their efforts mean they excel in what they do.

In today's fast-paced world, such an unambitious goal as 'act normal' may seem ludicrous, but in the context of niksen it is more relevant than ever. It implies that life is not so much about the flash and dash, a top-notch career and making money; it is about spending your time meaningfully. It may be one of the reasons why so many people in the Netherlands want to work part-time. It's not that they don't find work important, but they also prioritise time spent with their family and friends, charity work and having enough downtime to themselves.

Think of how you want to be remembered – as the person who would answer every email within the hour, or as a loving partner, great parent and loyal friend? Today more than ever you can decide how to live your life. It's up to you to design it.

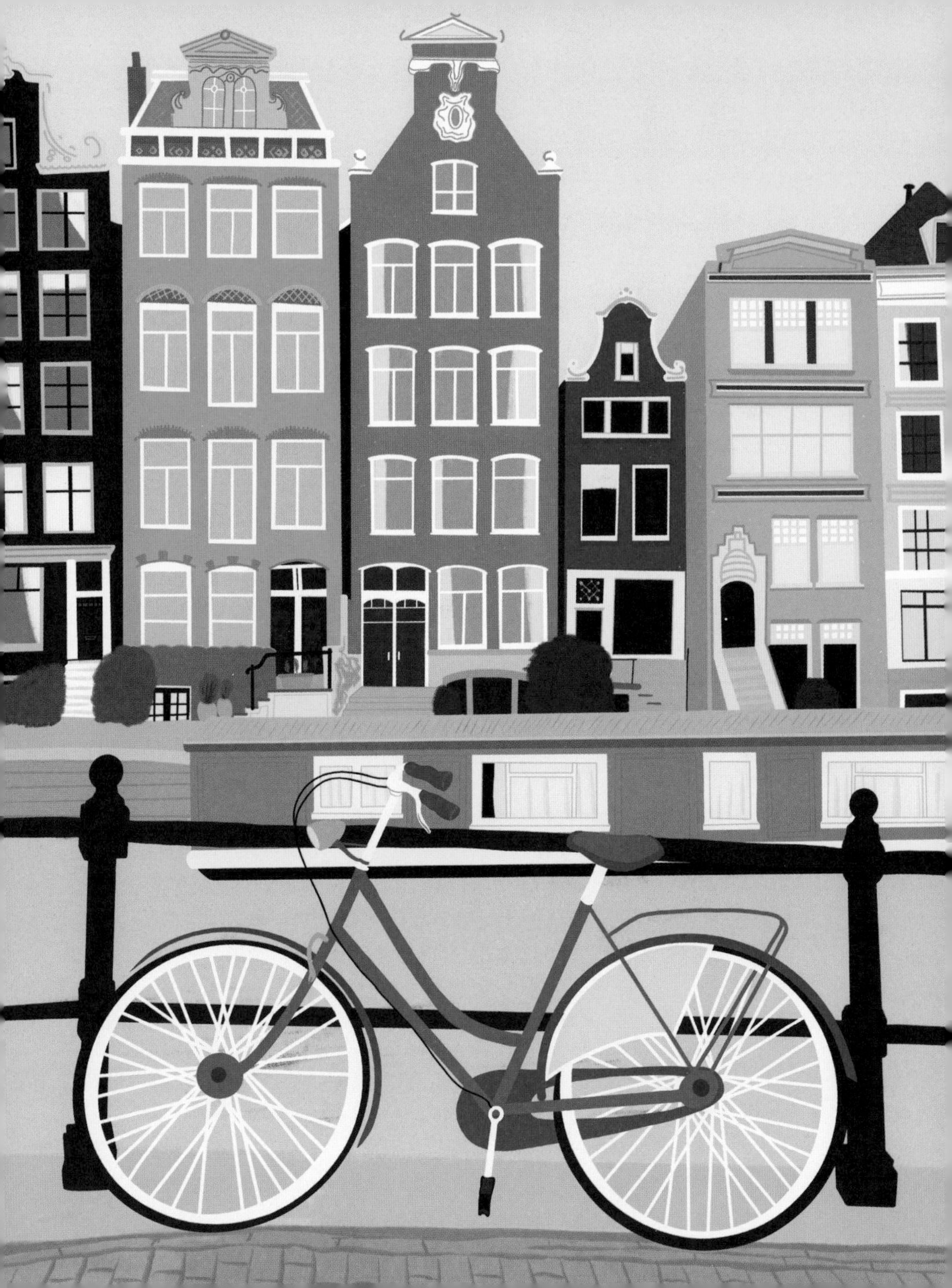

What Do You Care About?

Without giving it much thought, how would you answer this question? Researcher Wieteke Conen from the University of Amsterdam compared the values of Dutch people with the priorities of those from five other countries: United Kingdom, Germany, Italy, Czech Republic and Denmark.[1] And the results speak volumes...

All countries considered family the most important. But when it came to work, the Netherlands ranked this much lower than its neighbouring countries – after family, friends and free time. In most other countries, work came second. Of all six countries, workers in the Netherlands attached more value to free time than workers in any other country.

Free time is a priority we must all adopt. You may not have the luxury of being able to work fewer hours or take long holidays, but you can organise your time in a way that works for you. What do you need to feel balanced and whole? Is it professional accomplishment and financial success, your family, a vibrant social life; or is it health, wellbeing and personal development? This answer will help to determine what you see as a desirable work–life balance. You need to stop and take stock.

---

1 *Conen used data from the European Values Study (1981–2017), which offers insights into the aspects of work that Europeans value most and the importance they attach to work compared to other areas in their life.*

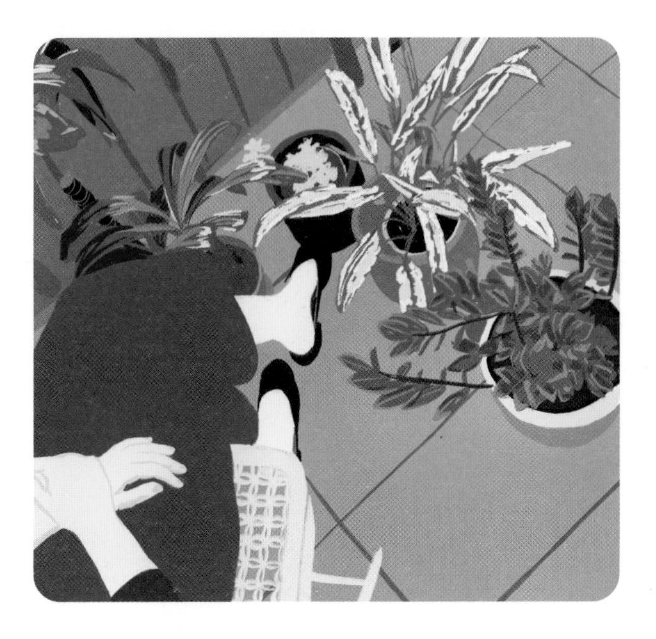

The Pleasure of Anticipation

Simply adding your niksen moment or day off to the calendar can increase your enjoyment of all the moments beforehand. The Dutch have a word for this, *voorpret*, meaning 'the joyful anticipation derived from imagining a future pleasure'. It's the reason why many Dutch people like to book their summer holiday in early January; it gives them something to look forward to in the cold and dark months that are still ahead. Psychologists have shown that the anticipation of positive events may indeed increase our overall satisfaction with life.

EXERCISE

KEEP A HAPPINESS DIARY

Find out for yourself what makes you happy with a daily review. Write a list of everything you did yesterday and, using a scale of 1 to 10, rate how happy these made you feel. Repeat this for several days or weeks to help you to make better choices and find a lifestyle that truly suits you. For example:

Get up	*7.0*
Eat	*7.5*
Work	*5.5*
Watch TV	*7.0*
Read a book	*8.0*
Exercise	*8.0*
On the road	*4.5*
Take a nap	*8.0*
Social media	*6.5*
Go to bed	*7.5*

The Happiness Diary will show if you are spending your time on the right things. If something consistently scores a 5.5 or less, it may be time for a change. Ring-fence free hours for activities you enjoy by not working overtime too often and taking a proper lunch break each day.[2] This exercise helps you gain an understanding of how you (want to) spend your time, and to carve out more moments of personal downtime.

---

2 *This exercise was inspired by De Gelukswijzer (gelukswijzer.nl), an online scientific study by the Erasmus Universiteit Rotterdam.*

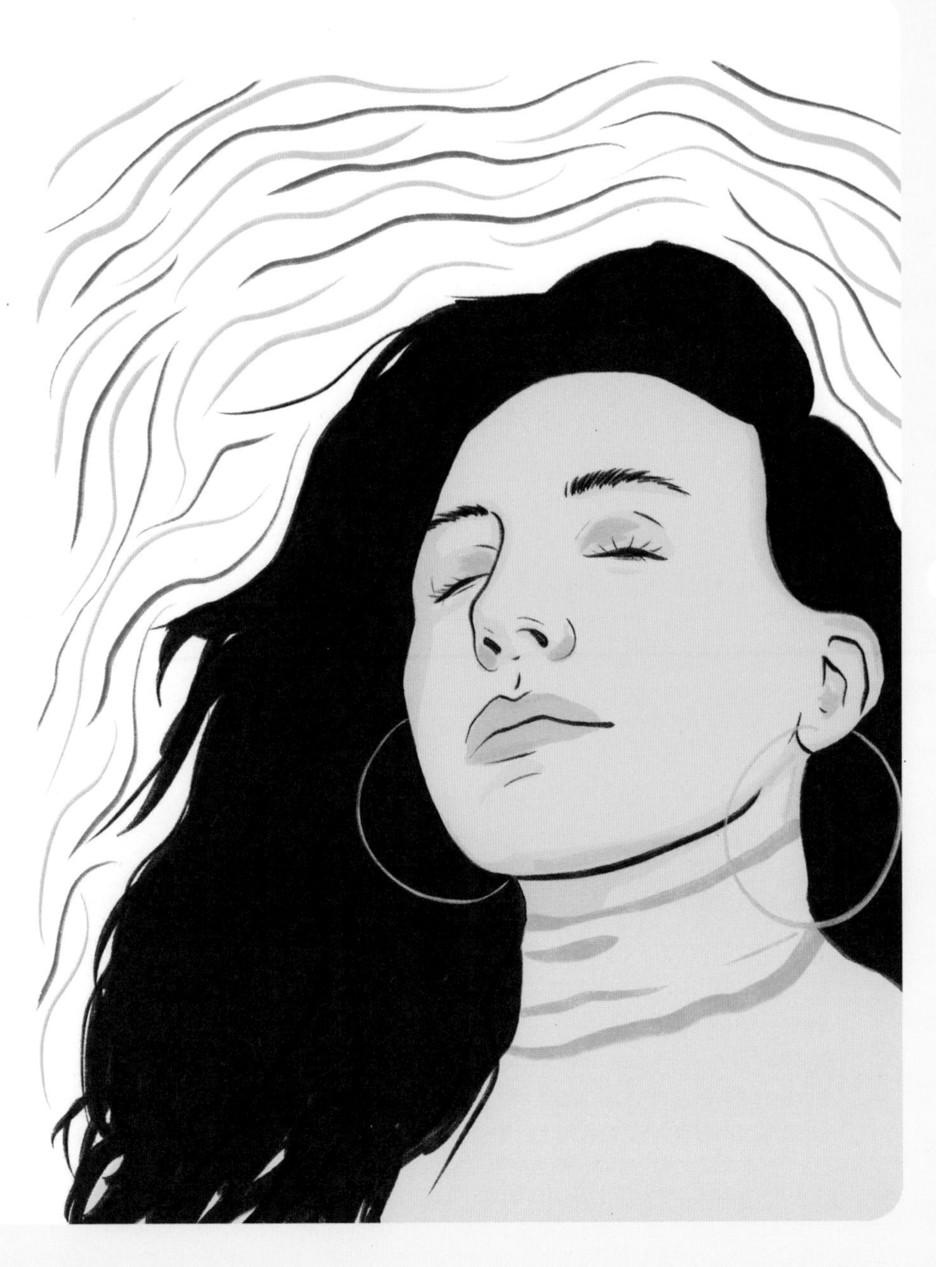

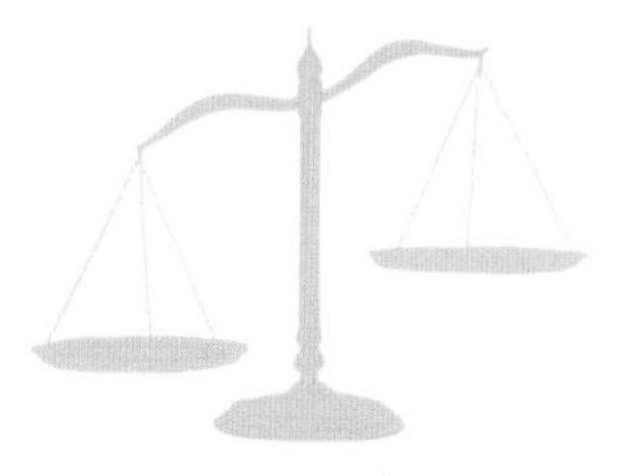

It's All About Balance

A life in which we are either busy all the time, or do absolutely nothing all day, lacks essential rhythm. A healthy and well-functioning brain needs both *ups and downs*; the contrasts between doing and not doing. You could compare it to the rhythmic pattern of the sea, the constant rising and falling motion of the waves.

Our brain is set up to deal with fluctuations in stress, constantly adapting to our daily challenges. Problems arise only if we don't allow ourselves timeouts to rest and recuperate, and the stress becomes chronic.

The state we want to reach is an organic flow of exertion and relaxation; our mind is active and engaged most of the time, but we have solid breaks away from it all. Ride that wave, but don't deny yourself the opportunity to regain strength in the calm waters of low tide. Your body and mind need that contraction, that time to rest, restore and reflect.

EXERCISE

RESTORATIVE BREATHING

Close your eyes and visualise the rhythmic pattern of the sea, following the rising and falling motion of the waves. Try to align your breathing with the movement. Imagine there's a wave coming whenever you breathe in, expanding your belly, then slowly breathe out to release. The waves may be messy at first, but as your breathing slows, the tide gradually becomes calmer.

Use this exercise as a quick pick-me-up on a busy day. You can do this anywhere – even on a bathroom break or behind your computer.

EXERCISE

MARKER TEST

Use this simple exercise to set your priorities for the week.

Write down all the things you plan to do this week, both professionally and personally. Now take a black marker and cross through all the things that can be postponed, delegated or cancelled. Only the most important tasks and activities can stay, a daily niksen break being one of them.

EXERCISE

THE HOUSE TEST

Imagine your life as a house, where each room represents a different aspect: work, family, play, health . . . and so on. Draw your house blueprints on a piece of paper to help you visualise it. Let's make it a typical Dutch house, with big windows (and no curtains) to allow the sunshine in.

The **bedroom** is where you sleep at least seven to eight hours per night.

The **home office** represents when and how you work.

Your **kitchen** may represent the time you spend with your family, where you nourish them and sit down at the table to help your kids with their homework.

The **bathroom** is the ideal space for self-care.

The **living room** could symbolise your social life: the place where you sit with your friends, dance and play, with quieter spaces for intimate conversations.

Assign a **separate niksen room** where you can reflect, dream and do nothing. (For more on how to create a niksen room in your actual home, see page 83).

The reality check

Now apply this house metaphor to your own life. Are you living in the house of your dreams – a nurturing place where you feel confident, supported and motivated? Think of the areas that matter to you most. Are you spending enough time in these spaces?

You may be spending too much time in your home office because you've been working overtime, or because your co-workers keep calling you at night and weekends. The few hours of free time you have left are used for family and friends, at the expense of time spent in your niksen room, which has remained unvisited for days.

Boundaries and self-care

Erect an invisible boundary around yourself; between yourself and the wave of people and things that threaten your space. A loving circle of friends brings an uplifting energy, but don't let in those with draining or toxic energies that disrespect your work hours. Don't take on tasks you can't manage. Creating space and establishing boundaries is important to maintaining your physical and mental health. Take care of yourself every day: listen to your gut when it's saying STOP, schedule enough time to nurture your soul, and spend time in your niksen room (see opposite).

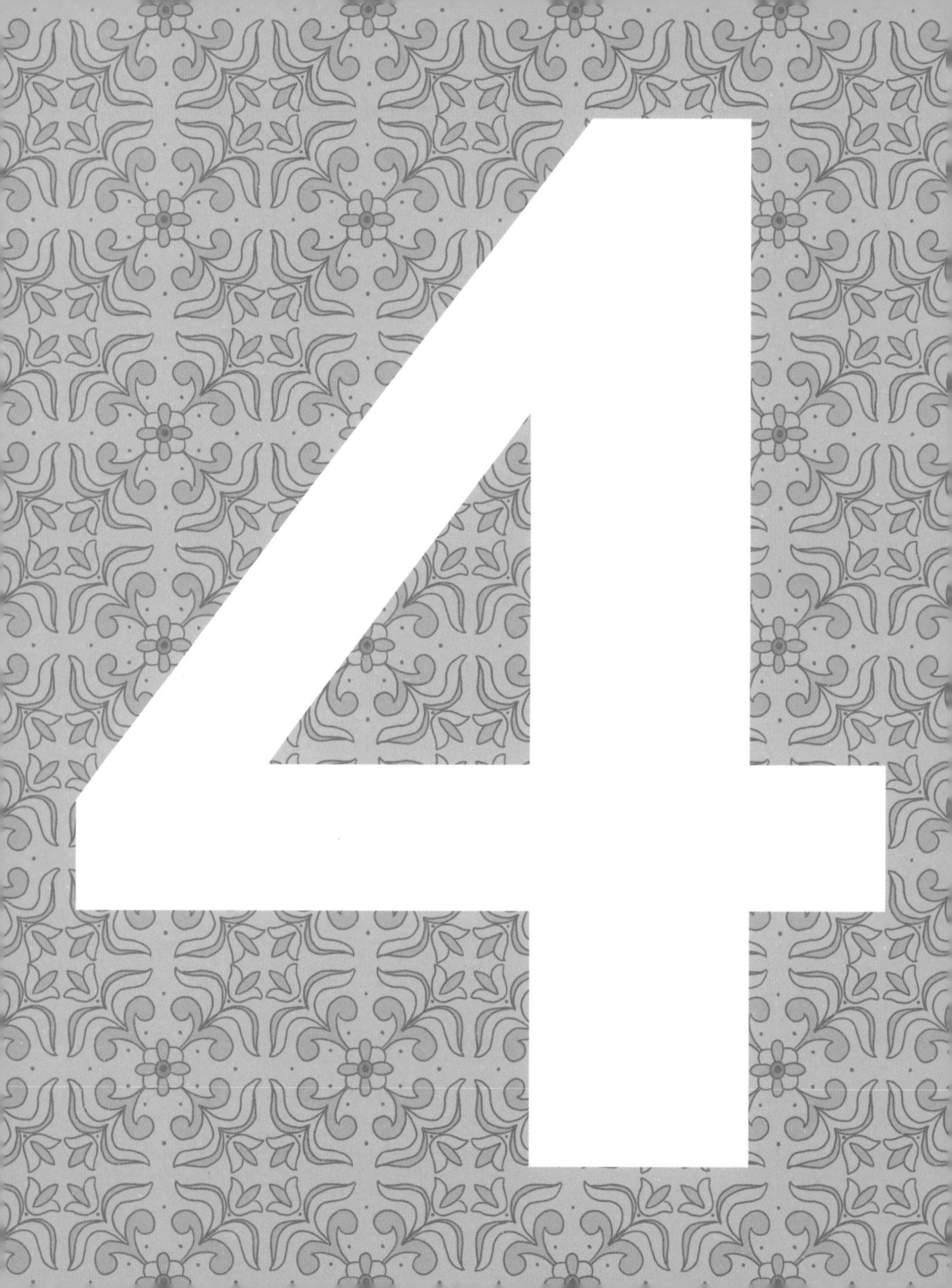
4

NIKSEN EVERY DAY

Work, children, exercise, social gatherings ... your week may fill up faster than tables at the world's best restaurant! In this chapter we will look at ways of creating more physical and mental space for doing nothing. Time is a precious commodity because it can only be spent once. So we need to allocate the hours in our days as wisely as possible, dividing them between time spent on things we have to do and the moments when we can simply be.

Living on Dutch Time

When I'm very busy, I sometimes long for the Sundays of my youth. In the town where I lived, this day of the week used to be a collective moment of rest and laziness. The shops were closed, most people had the day off, and there would be little to no traffic in the streets. Time seemed to slow itself, offering a proper break. No matter how busy the week, you knew you would have Sunday off to rest and be lazy.

Today it's not the church or state but ourselves who decide when we work and rest; we can shop around the clock, and seek distraction whenever things are too quiet for our liking. The number of hours we have in a day remains unaltered, but the amount of activities we cram into those 24 hours, seven days a week, has increased massively, and sometimes it seems as though we've become addicted to being busy all the time. If most of your Sundays feel like Tuesdays and you want this madness to stop, niksen is for you.

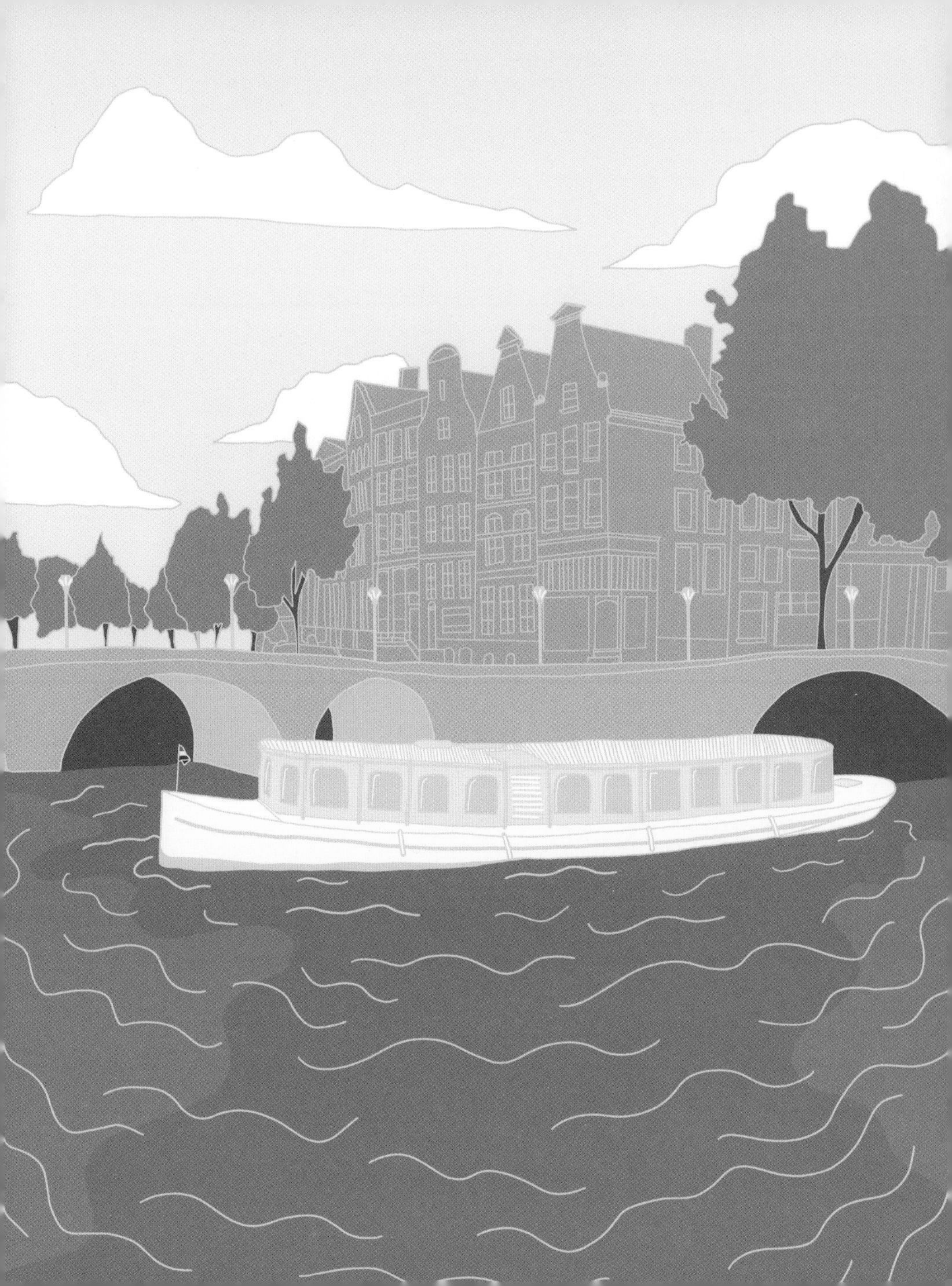

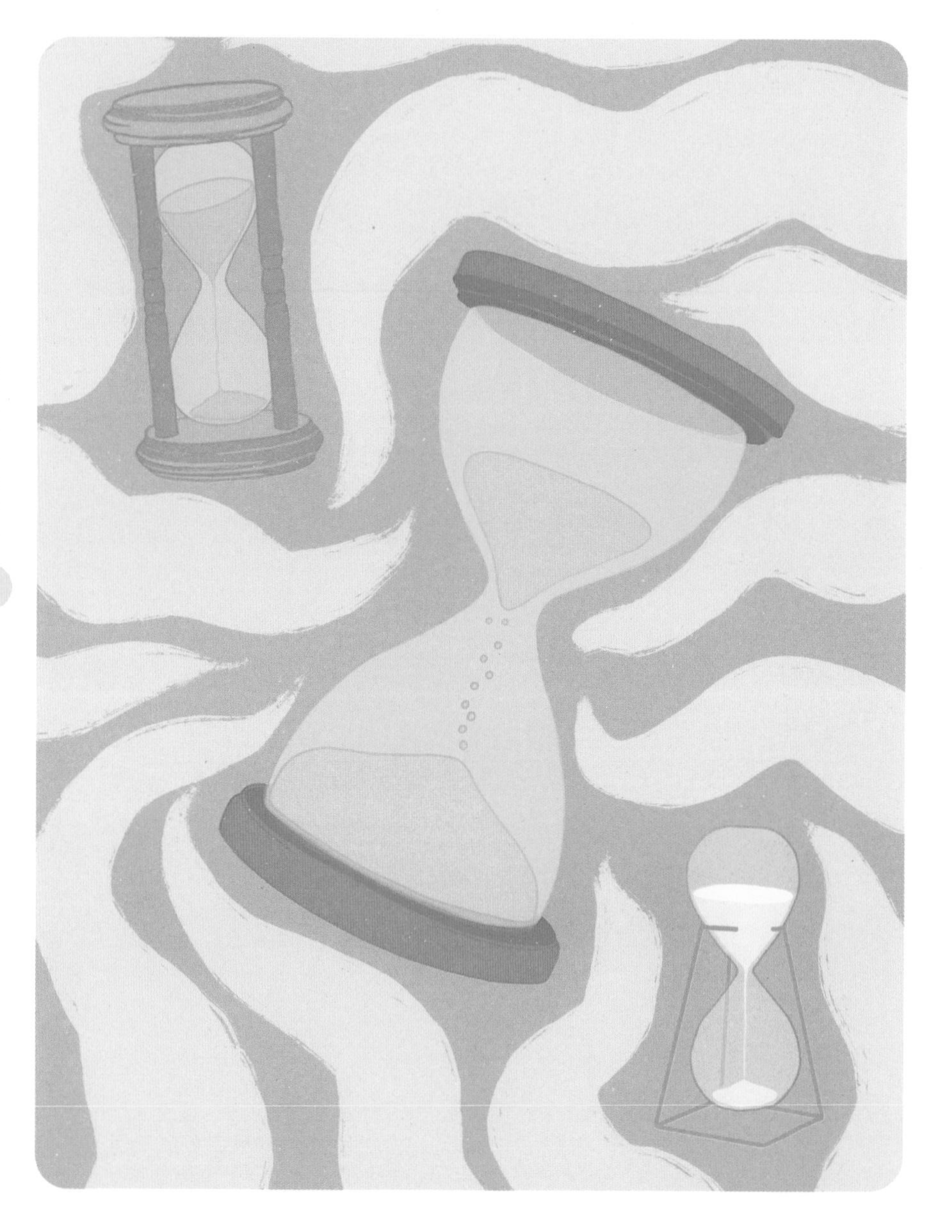

How to say no, the Dutch way

In the Netherlands, the trait of truthfulness comes before empathy. Just as many Dutch would share their opinion about your new clothes or give you honest feedback about your work, they will also tell you directly if they can't meet your request, or simply don't feel like it. Whereas others would denounce this straightforwardness as blunt or even rude, it is not intended that way.

Do you want to cancel a dinner date because you need some time to yourself? Just say so. It's okay, you can still be friends. In fact, the other person would probably do the same thing.

The Dutch and scheduling

Dutch people love their pocket planners and digital diaries. In the Netherlands, showing up at someone's doorstep unannounced can lead to an awkward situation. Coffee dates are seldom on impulse, and a get-together with friends is planned weeks ahead.

This is *overzichtelijkheid*, the joy of scheduling, bringing order to the chaos and making the week more predictable and manageable. If you find out on Monday that you have a work presentation on Thursday, you will need to block out a few hours on Wednesday to prepare. And scheduling can also be used to protect your free time, and even to create windows for niksen. After all, if you already use a planner for your work meetings and doctor appointments, why wouldn't you do the same for something as essential as your personal downtime?

Niksen in Your Everyday Routine

There is a time for work, a time for family and friends, and a time for relaxation. Organise your days to allow space for all of these, as too much of any one thing will cause an imbalance and undue stress.

How much free time do we need?

If we're too busy to spend time on the things that matter most, we can become chronically stressed, depleted of energy and unsatisfied. On the other hand, too much free time can be mind-numbing, leading to feelings of boredom and dissatisfaction. We can also feel lonely if we have more free time than the people surrounding us.

So how much free time do we need to be at our happiest? A 2018 study by the University of Pennsylvania and the UCLA[1] suggests that 2.5 hours a day, for people who work full-time, is optimal. Less than that and most people feel stressed. More than that and they feel lazy and unproductive. Personality will also play a part – some people may need more free time than others. The ideas opposite will help you to schedule your niksen moments, and allow you to judge how much time works for you.

---

1 *Sharif, Marissa and Mogilner, Cassie and Hershfield, Hal, 'The Effects of Being Time Poor and Time Rich on Life Satisfaction' (November 15, 2018).*

Making your calendar work for niksen

Make niksen a priority. Block out around 20 minutes every workday and two hours a day at the weekend. Don't be too fixated on the exact duration though; the key thing is to plan a timeout every day.

Schedule specific amounts of time. Plan for how long you expect to spend on your tasks. If you finish before the allotted time, use this as a window of opportunity to do nothing.

Be realistic and stringent. You should be able to accomplish all the activities you've put into your calendar. If you have to cross out niksen because of an unforeseen event, move it to another time.

Allow time between tasks for unexpected delays, spontaneous events, or simply to do nothing at all. This space can also protect you from having to do work in the evenings or at weekends.

Schedule time for a weekly review. If you don't stop every now and then to look at the bigger picture, you'll end up playing catch-up and forget about your planned timeouts.

Categorise different types of event. Use different-coloured labels, and you'll see at a glance if you're dividing your time in a balanced way. Then you can fix things accordingly.

Drop anchors in your calendar

Imagine you have an entire weekend completely to yourself, to do whatever you want. Sounds like heaven, right? The reality might be a little different. A whole weekend with no direction often leaves us restless and indecisive; this boundless space, with hours of endless possibilities, can feel overwhelming and anything but relaxing. In this situation, niksen will become something negative.

'Time has purpose and meaning only if it's being structured by a rhythm, with a recognisable and recurring pattern,' says philosopher Marli Huijer.[2] Now, imagine you're working until 5pm and will meet a friend at 8pm. Your schedule suddenly has a defined space to use as you please, long enough to not feel rushed, but short enough to not feel lost.

Whenever you need a reminder of the need for structure and routine, picture the famous dikes of the Netherlands. Just as they define the space where the Dutch can live and thrive, and protect the land from flooding, the anchors you drop in your calendar help define the space you spend on niksen, and protect you from feeling overwhelmed.

---

2 *'Zoeken naar het juiste ritme in de 24-uurs economie' ['Finding the right rhythm in the 24-hour economy'],* Filosofie Magazine, *2008.*

EXERCISE

TIME WELL SPENT?

Create time for a weekly review. Find a comfortable spot that's not your desk. Once you're settled, start by writing down anything that's currently on your mind. This will allow you to put your issues to one side and help you focus more clearly on the exercise (see 'mental minimalism', page 81). Take ten minutes to relax and create some distance from your everyday stuff; you can doodle, stare out of the window or close your eyes.

Once you feel more relaxed, ask yourself three simple questions:

Am I happy with what I have achieved this week?

Did I take as many timeouts as I had planned to?

What can I do in the upcoming week to make my timeouts happen?

Your answers will reveal whether you've let your deadlines interfere with the time spent on nothing, and will help you set your intentions for the week ahead.

Niksen Anytime

Some days it can be hard to find space for a quiet, gentle moment, because time is simply not on your side. But even if you have only a brief window, try to take a breather from your obligations and turn inwards. If the idea of niksen makes you feel awkward or downright uncomfortable, take baby steps. Be patient and start with a few minutes each day, until you have got used to the idea of doing nothing, then gradually expand this to half an hour or more each day.

Niksen if you have ...

○ **No time at all**

Squeeze a stress ball. The great thing is that you can do this anywhere – while sitting at your desk, or even when you're in a meeting. Squeezing the ball activates the muscles in your hand and wrist, and releasing your grip allows them to relax, alleviating tension and stress.

5 minutes

Clear desk, clear mind! Tidy away anything in your immediate vicinity that isn't needed today. The benefits are twofold: the task of cleaning can be a soothing, rewarding therapy in its own right, and the result is a more calming environment to niks in. Win-win.

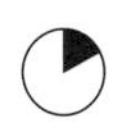

10 minutes

Take a moment to envision yourself in a place where you feel content and relaxed, to provide your brain with positive suggestions that counterbalance stressful emotions. Close your eyes and recall all the details, from the scents and sounds to the colours and beautiful sights that are enveloping you. Use all your senses to bring your happy place to life in your mind's eye until you are fully immersed in it, helping you reach a blissful state of niksen.

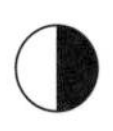

30 minutes

Progressive muscle relaxation awakens your body and mind and loosens muscles that get tight from sitting or standing all day. Find a relaxed position (seated or lying down) and tune into your body. Tighten a muscle and then release it, working from your feet all the way up to your head. Close your eyes and feel the tension flowing out of your body.

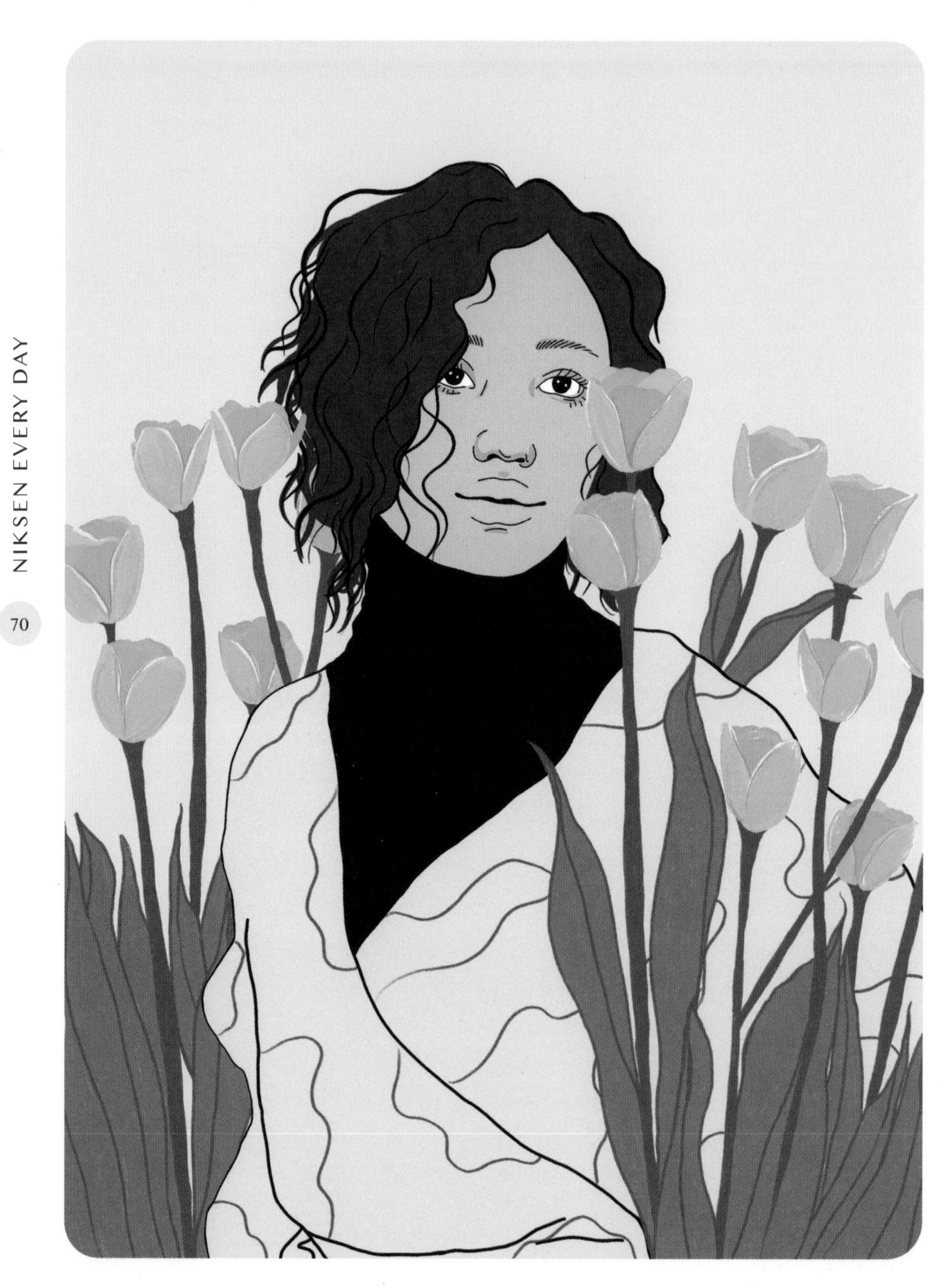

Protect Your Timeout

Prevent yourself and others from bulldozing over your carefully scheduled downtime. If you are honest about your personal needs, you are putting your best interests first – and what could be wrong with that?

Be more direct

Be more Dutch and don't be afraid to say no. The other person may be disappointed at first, but at least they know where they stand. Just make sure you choose your words carefully, so things don't get awkward.

- **Be candid.**
  If someone is asking for a favour, you can simply say, 'Sorry, today I can't.' And be honest about your constraints: 'I've been so busy lately that I had planned some much-needed time for myself.' Don't try and come up with a list of reasons why you can't meet their request, as these may come across as lame excuses.

- **Keep it simple.**
  If you don't want to go into detail, simply say: 'Sadly, I'm afraid I can't help you with that.' You're acknowledging that your answer might disappoint the recipient and that it brings you no joy to say no.

- **Keep your options open.**
  You could add: 'I can't right now, but please keep me in mind for future assignments/events.' Your *no* doesn't mean they can't ask you again in the future, it simply means that right now you're unable to help.

- **Say no in person.**
  Messaging is one of the most notorious sources of misinterpretation. Call the other person or, if they are in the same office, quickly drop by so they can hear your tone of voice and see your facial expression and body language. Never become defensive or aggressive; show them it's nothing personal, just something that you cannot do right now.

Ask for help

Be proactive and let people know if you are struggling to get your work done on time. Don't jeopardise your free time, but instead ask your co-workers or a friend for help. They can take over some of your work tasks, or collect your kids from the nursery so you get an extra hour. They will probably be happy to help, and if not, they will say so (if they're smart).

A Dutch person would advise you:

'*Nee heb je, ja kun je krijgen*'

(literally: 'You have a no, a yes you can get'), which essentially means 'It doesn't hurt to ask.'

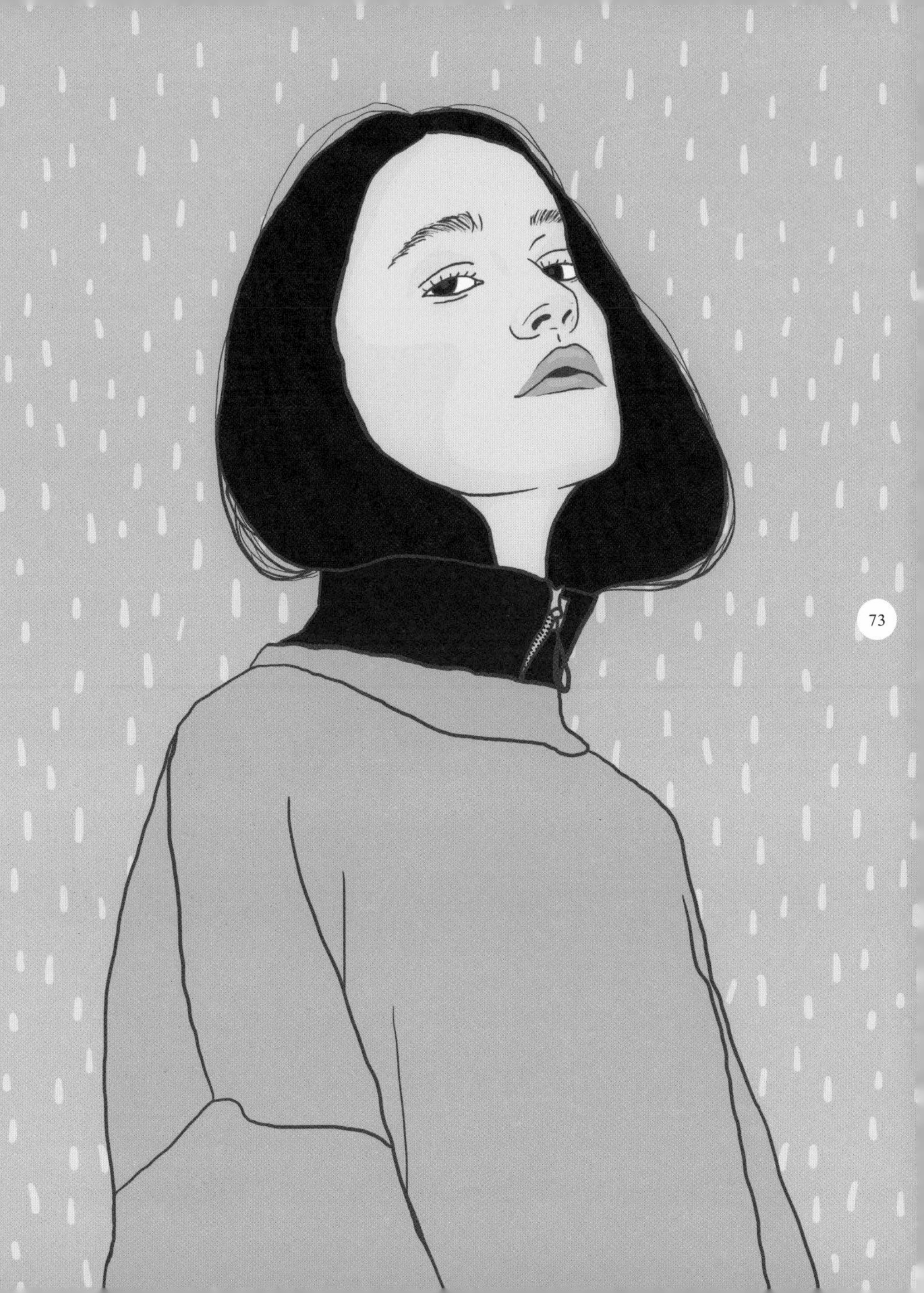

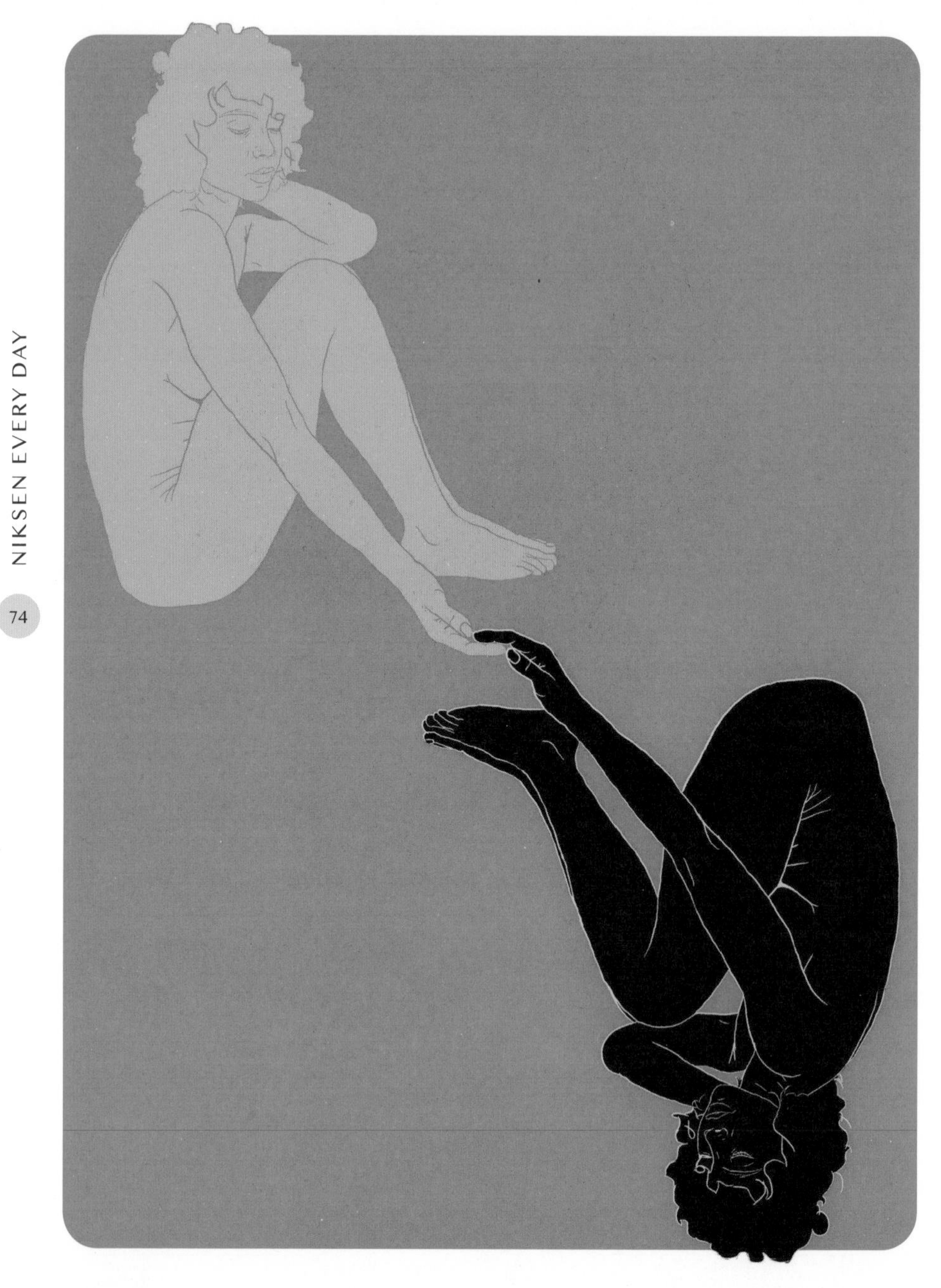

Don't feel intimidated

There will come a time when someone sees you doing nothing and asks, with a somewhat ironic tone, 'Are you having a good time?' or, more straightforwardly, 'Don't you have anything better to do?' Don't make up excuses; be frank and simply tell them that you're doing nothing because you feel like it. Keep in mind that anyone who reacts this way is probably having a hard time unwinding themselves. You may want to show them this book to help them master the skill of niksen.

Help yourself

Sometimes it's not others who threaten our timeout, but the voices in our own head. Can't resist thinking about work and other obligations, even in your free time? Mute your phone, switch off your notifications and try to turn your attention elsewhere. In Chapter 7 (see page 122) we look at ways to relax your mind, without pushing it.

Wish others their own timeout

Keep negativity at bay by wishing others their own timeout. Create a culture where niksen is not an uncommon occurrence or a random treat, but a necessity and a sign of respect. Encourage colleagues to take a proper lunch break to allow them to recharge. Do the same at home: cook dinner for your housemate if they work late, check in with your partner or child to see if they are overwhelmed and need anything. See page 30 for more on the Dutch skill of generosity, *gunnen*, and how to pay it forward.

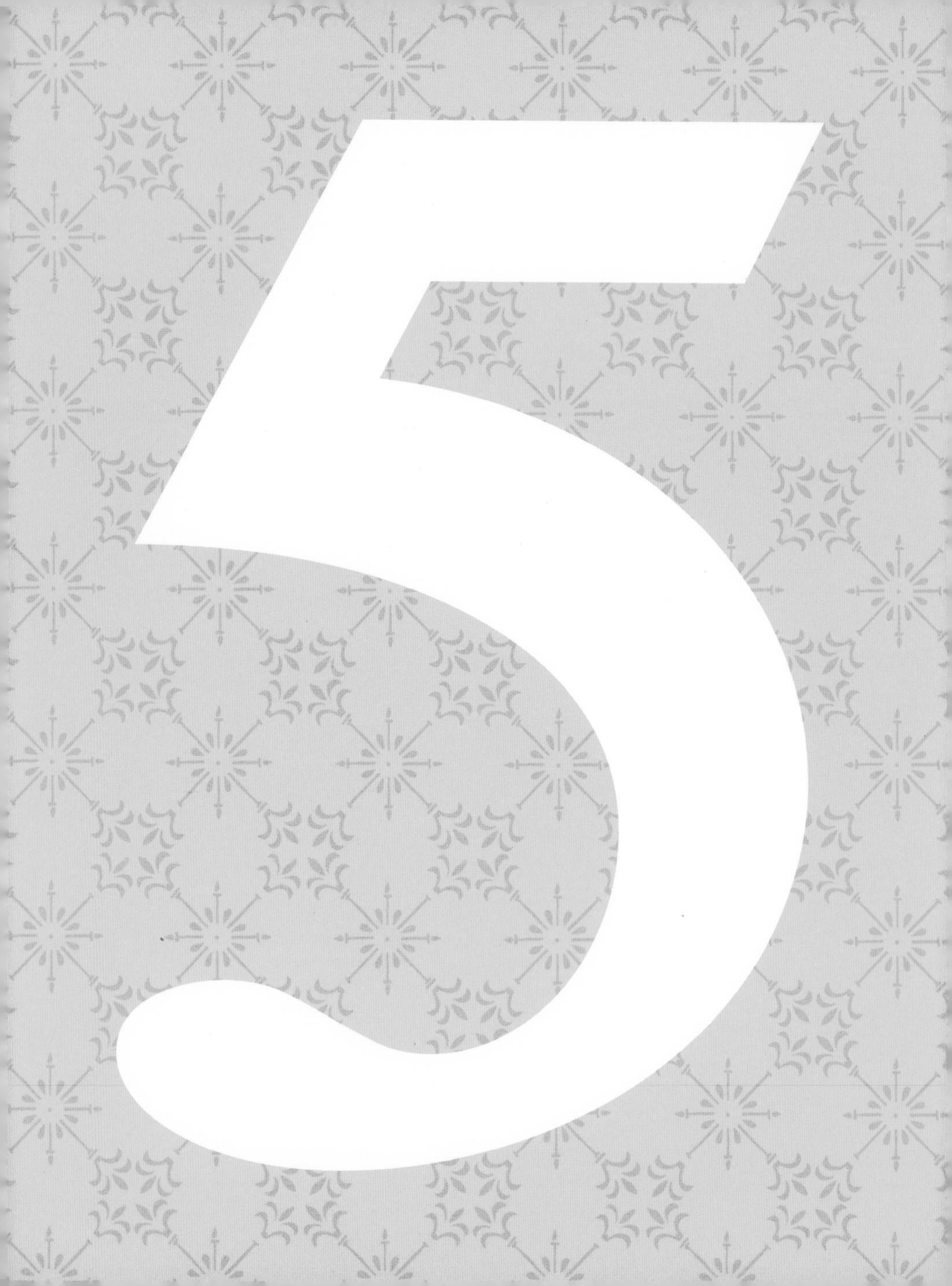

NIKSEN ANYWHERE

In the previous chapter we talked about the when. Here, we get into the where: how you can bring niksen into your home, workplace, holiday and even online. You'll learn how to make any environment into a niksen sanctuary by focusing your mind on the right things, and addressing and removing any obstacles in your way.

Niksen at Home

It can be tricky to carve out time to do nothing within the confines of your own home. Before you know it, your carefully scheduled me-time has been swallowed by all kinds of domestic chores and life admin. Sometimes the problem is not that we don't have enough downtime, but that we don't use it mindfully.

Many of us have a hard time disconnecting at home, and by Sunday night we're already tense because we know we need to work again the next morning. We're so obsessed with the clock and our to-do lists that we find ourselves swimming in thoughts that have a talent for lodging inside our head and repeating on an endless loop. Maybe we don't need more hours of free time, but simply to treat the downtime we do have with more awareness, ridding ourselves of mental clutter.

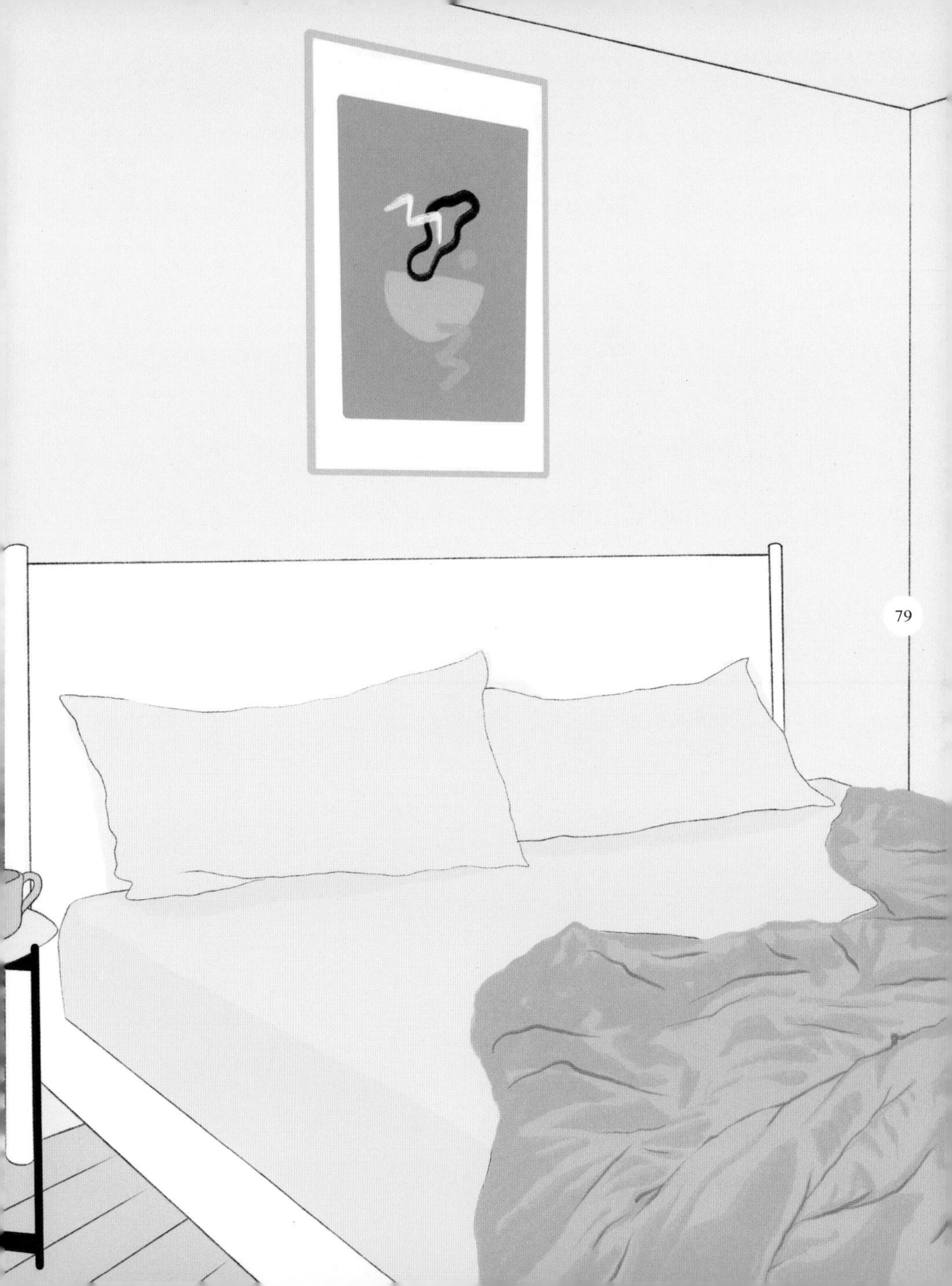

EXERCISE

WAKE UP WITH NIKSEN

First thing in the morning is a golden time to niks. The world is quiet and half-asleep. Your eyes blink open and your mind is clear, unfogged by the stresses of the day. Sit up and look out of the window. Let your mind wander, and breathe slowly in and out. Make this a sacred morning ritual and remember these three no-nos:

①

DO NOT be tempted to shut your eyes and go back to sleep.

②

DO NOT grab your phone as soon as you are conscious (keep this outside your bedroom if possible).

③

DO NOT reach for the TV remote or switch on any other device, to check your emails, social media or the news.

Clean out your mental space

A lack of mental space means you have no room to fully engage in a conversation or an experience because your mind is already at capacity. Use the following strategies to create more headspace and start using your home (and downtime) as it should be used: to retreat, disconnect and recuperate.

Mental minimalism

Our head can sometimes feel like an internet browser that has more tabs open than can fit on the screen. Don't keep everything stored in your brain. Instead, write it down. Find an app or a notebook and jot down any thoughts, tips, tasks or links you want to bookmark for later.

If your timeout is constantly interrupted by internal chatter, write down your worries and concerns. Treat your journal as a private space where you can be totally frank with yourself. Putting your words on paper helps to get things off your chest, allowing you to see things in perspective and even to find a solution. Recognise what you are in control of and cross out anything that's out of your hands.

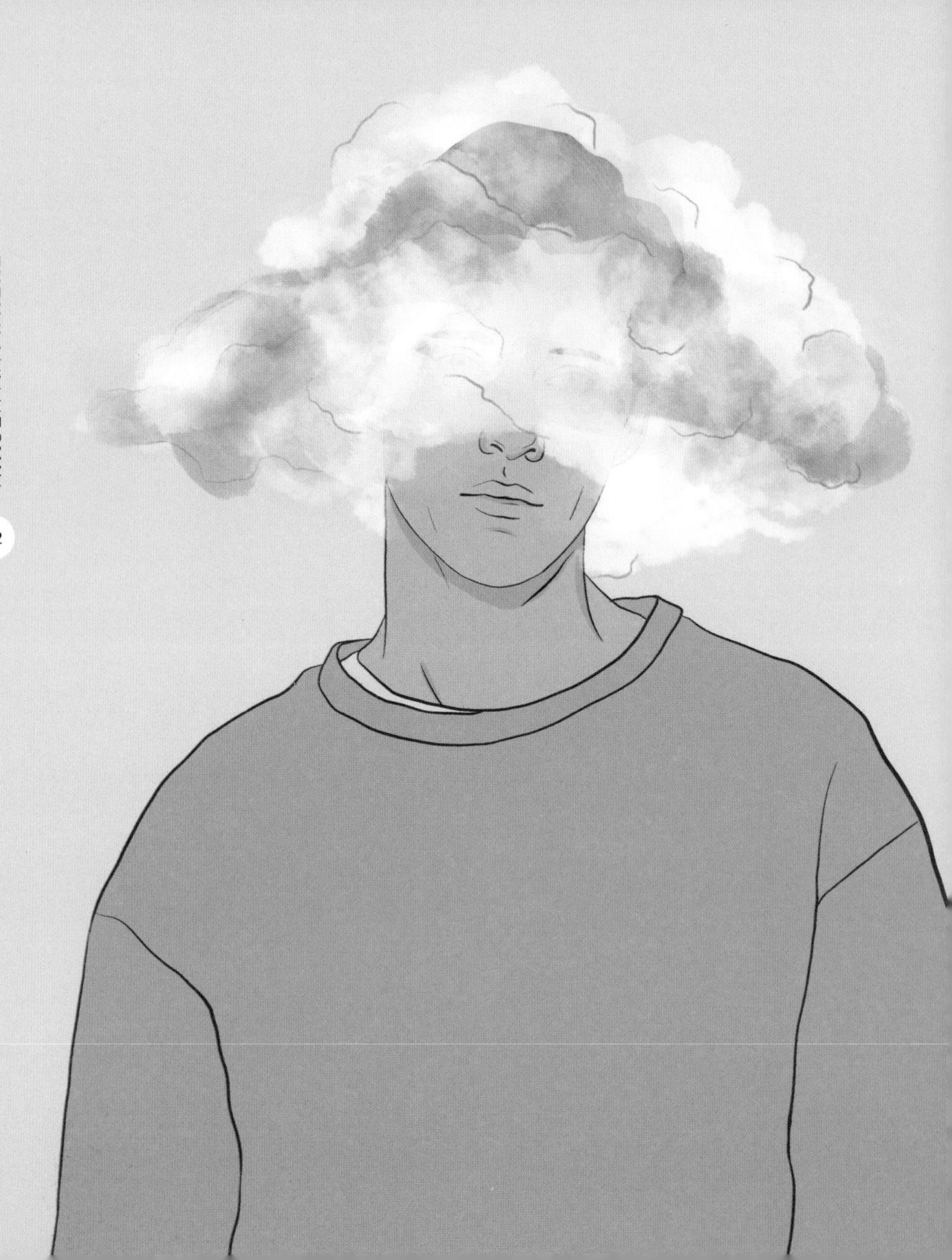

Declutter your physical environment

Excessive stimuli force your brain to work overtime, signalling that there's always something else that needs to be done, distracting you and endangering your timeout. Declutter all the spaces that you may retreat to for doing nothing, such as the living room, bedroom and bathroom, keeping only the essential stuff and organising the rest so it can easily be found and accessed when needed.

Create a Niksen Sanctuary, Dutch-style

If you have young kids running around, it may seem like a non-starter to keep the communal spaces of your house decluttered. To help with this, identify at least one area in the house as your niksen space. If you don't have a spare room or shed to retreat to, find a window seat or use a corner of your bedroom and claim it as your own.

Make this space as cosy, pleasant and *gezellig* as possible (see page 22). Add a comfortable chair, bring some nature inside with a bunch of fresh flowers and turn off your phone. The trick to creating this worry-free zone is to make it your own and not to overload it with unnecessary clutter. This is your sanctuary, where you can safely turn inwards and reflect. Fresh air and sunshine flow through the space, bringing creativity and clarity of mind.

Niksen in the Workplace

The *possibility* that we can be accessible always and everywhere has led to the *expectation* that we are accessible always and everywhere. Add to that the fact that more than ever we tend to identify ourselves with our job – which is assumed to be nothing less than our 'passion' – and the line between our professional and personal life is truly blurred. All at the expense of time to rest and revive ourselves.

We can't clone ourselves or add more hours to the day, but we can be smarter with the resources we have. The magical word here is 'boundaries'. Create physical distance between yourself and your office and be firm about what you can and cannot handle. And prioritise niksen to prioritise yourself: the amount of undisturbed time you allocate to it may sometimes be small, but what matters most is that you build and maintain a buffer between your obligations and your time out.

The following dos and don'ts will help you create more space between your professional and personal life, and in doing so carve out more opportunities to do nothing.

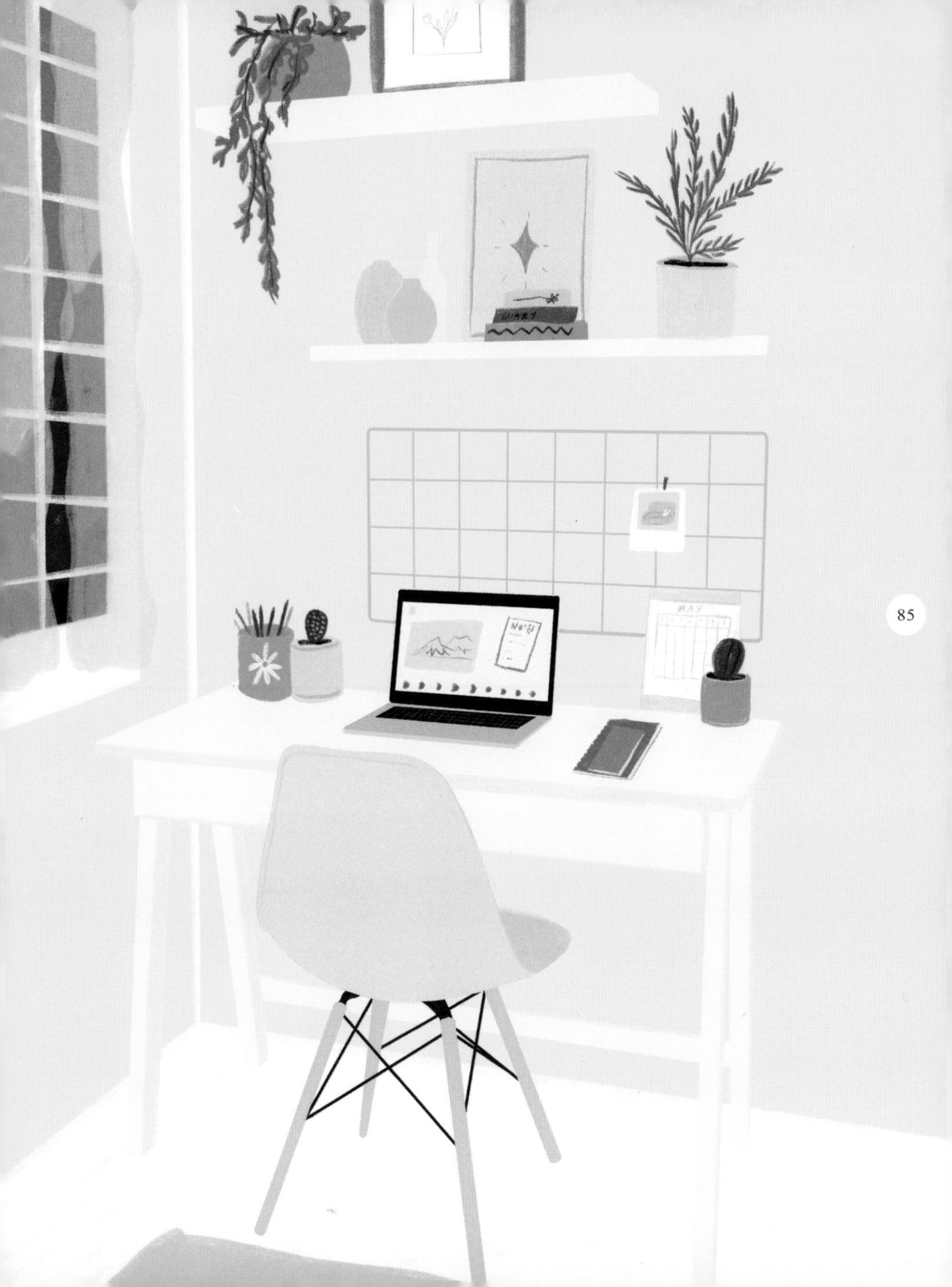
DIARY
MAY

Don't...

- Fill your week to the brim with work commitments. Be selective with the meetings you join: are they really useful for you, or can you join just for the relevant part?
- Spend more than two hours at your computer without taking a break.
- Multitask if you don't have to. Be fully present, whether at work, with your children or doing nothing.
- Take your laptop with you on a weekend getaway, or look at your phone during a lunch or dinner date.
- Say yes to Friday night drinks with your colleagues if you're tired and would prefer to go home. Nobody will blame you for taking care of yourself.
- Allow clients to call or text you outside office hours and expect an immediate response.
- Feel pressured to answer emails within an hour. People will call if there's an emergency.

Do...

- Designate specific times of day for dealing with emails. Close your mail server at all other times, and set up an automatic 'out of office' reply for weekends and holidays.
- Let clients and co-workers know if you don't want them to call you in the evenings or at weekends.
- Use an online conferencing service to schedule your calls, with a 24-hour advance notice to set up a meeting.
- Get out of your workplace and eat your lunch in a nearby park or another quiet spot, and be honest with your co-workers if you want to be alone.
- Turn your work phone off at home and at the weekend, and only use your personal phone (but don't share this number with your colleagues).
- Designate a space in the house as your home office. Your work items can be used in this room only.
- Use noise-blocking headphones and put your phone in flight mode if you need to focus.

Maximise your lunch break for niksen

It is vital that you don't skip your lunch break because you believe you have too much work waiting for you. The best way to stay focused throughout the day and increase your productivity is to give yourself a proper break and slow down for an hour. The following tips will help make your lunch hour one of the most relaxing events of the day, and the time you invest you will earn back in the afternoon.

- Start with a brief meditation or a relaxation exercise to quickly reset your body and mind. A newcomer in this field? Try the exercises on page 124. Once you feel more relaxed, take at least half an hour to do nothing, allowing your mind to go anywhere but your work projects. This time is yours to claim.

- Go for a walk at a relaxed pace. Research suggests this boosts brain function and mood, which can be handy if you have an important meeting planned for the afternoon.

- If you are fortunate enough to work close to a forest or a park, spend your lunch hour sitting on the grass or on a bench, savouring the soothing effects of nature. Watch how the sunlight is filtered through the canopy of trees, inhale the fresh forest air, close your eyes and listen to the birdsong and rustling of leaves. Even half an hour of forest bathing has reported benefits for our physiological, mental and emotional wellbeing.

- If there's no greenery near to your workplace, find a peaceful spot away from your desk that you can dedicate to some time out.

Productivity and niksen

If you (or your boss) fear that all this extra free time will jeopardise your productivity, listen up. Pilot tests of shorter work weeks show that fewer people call in sick, and that it doesn't have an adverse effect on productivity. In fact, those with less time at their disposal become more efficient and better at setting priorities. They achieve the same targets, with more opportunities to rest and relax. This corresponds with other studies which show that out of the usual eight hours in a workday, there are normally only three hours in which we are truly productive.

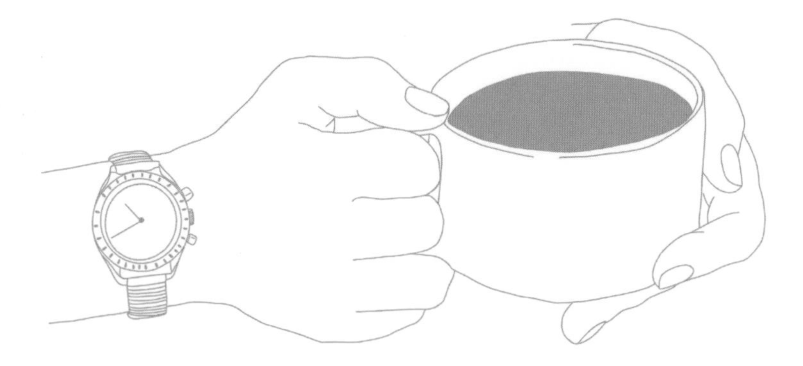

EXERCISE

GO POMODORO

To help me stay focused and productive through large work projects I use the Pomodoro technique, which was developed by the Italian time-management expert Francesco Cirillo.

①
Choose the task you want to complete today.

②
Set a kitchen timer or the timer on your phone for 25 minutes.
(Cirillo used a tomato-shaped timer, hence the name 'Pomodoro' technique, Italian for tomato).

③
Focus on the task and work uninterruptedly until the timer rings.

④
Take a break of five minutes, and spend it doing whatever you want as long as it's not work-related.

⑤
After four Pomodoros you can take a longer break, of 20 to 30 minutes.

I love this technique, because 25 minutes of work is long enough to be productive, yet short enough to not lose focus. And there is always the prospect of an upcoming timeout in sight.

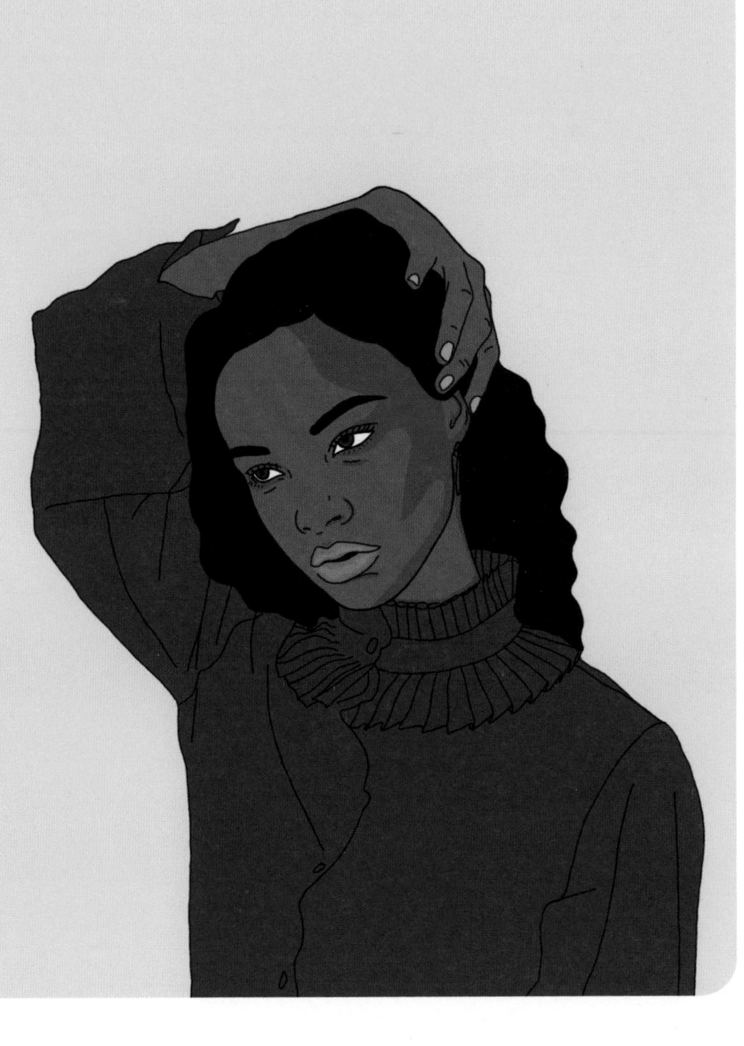

EXERCISE

EAT THE FROG

If you feel busy all day yet don't accomplish a single important task, you may be interested in Eat the Frog, a time-management method from self-development author Brian Tracy, which was inspired by a Mark Twain quote:

'If it's your job to eat a frog,
it's best to do it first thing in the morning.
And if it's your job to eat two frogs,
it's best to eat the biggest one first.'

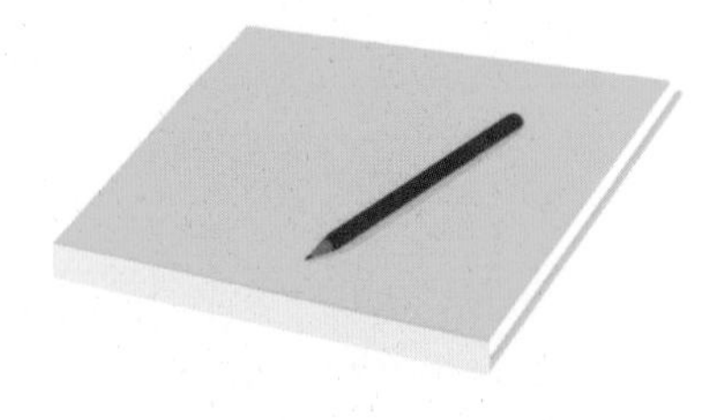

①

Identify the frog

Decide which task on your to-do list is something you don't want to do but you actually *need* to do. While you procrastinate on it, the task starts weighing on your mind, causing pressure and stress.

②

Eat it

Start working on the task without thinking too much about it and don't stop until it's finished.

③

Postpone nothing

Do this task first thing in the morning, when the office is still quiet, your mind is clearer and your willpower not yet depleted.

④

When there are two or more frogs

If there's more than one important thing to do during the day, tackle the biggest one first.

Once these problematic tasks are done, you will feel more satisfied and may use the momentum to tackle even more things. But keep this within a set timeframe. You are looking to work smarter, not harder. Add a niksen break between each task to keep your mind fresh and focused.

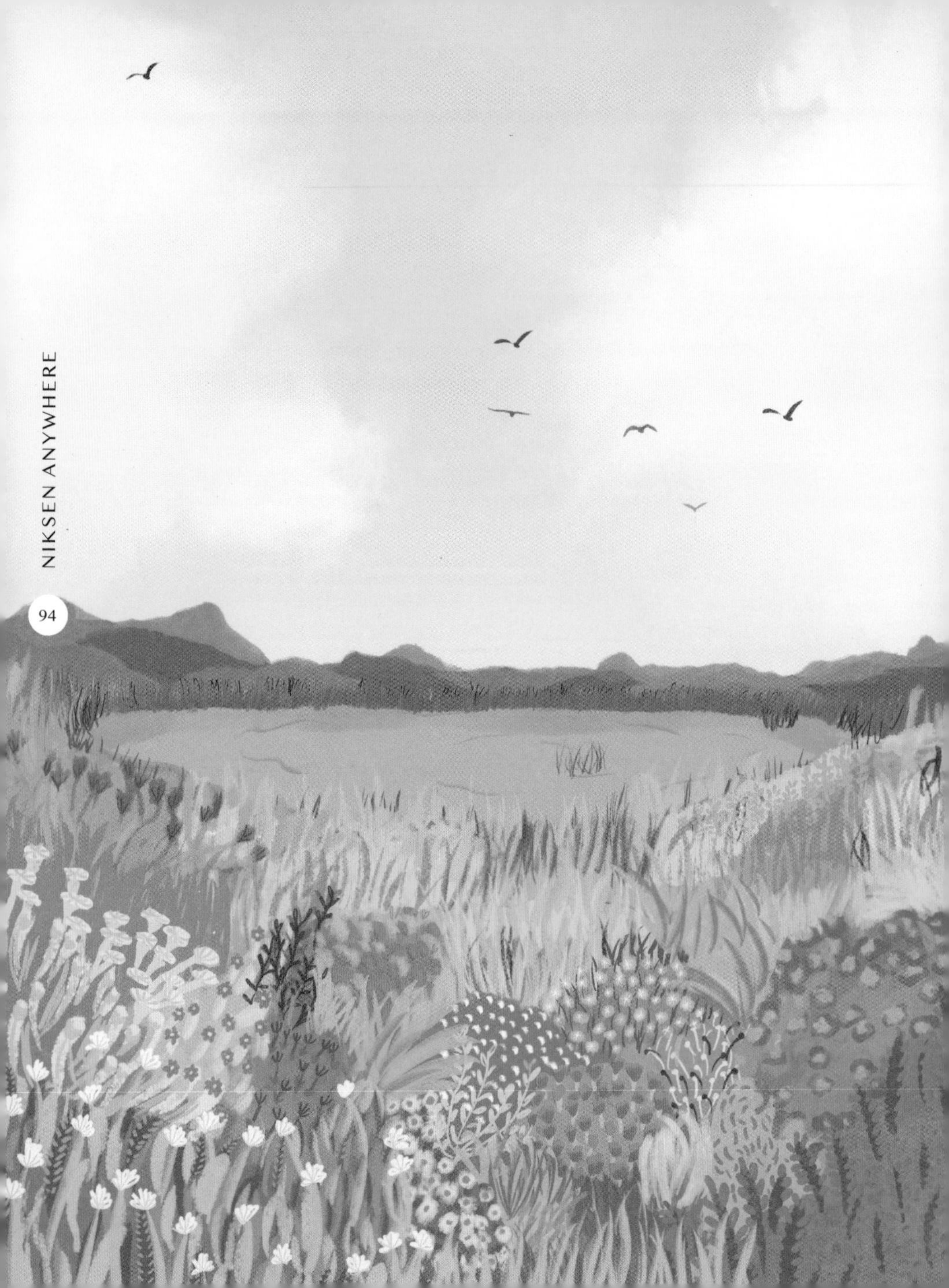

Niksen on Holiday

Finally, the day is here. Everything's organised.

You've booked a wonderful hotel for the week, with swimming pool and spa. It's going to be the most chilled holiday you've ever had, spending your days eating, reading and doing nothing. It's only once you've arrived that you realise how hard it is to unwind.

In practice, a one-week holiday often means only a couple of days of relaxation. It can take up to three days to wind down, and before the end of the week you will already be anticipating what you need to do when you get home.

Because of this, many companies in the Netherlands make it mandatory for their employees to take at least one 14-day period of leave every year.

While you may not be able to take two weeks off, the following suggestions will help you get into the right state of mind as quickly as possible.

Do only what's necessary before you leave

Do you usually want to empty your inbox, triple check if your co-workers know what to do during your absence, and clean out the dishwasher before you pull the door behind you? Then remind yourself that you'll be back in a week. Do what you can, but *goed is goed* ('good is good enough'). Pat yourself on the back and let yourself unwind.

Disconnect from home

If you want to take your phone with you, and maybe even your laptop, temporarily delete your mail application and social media. This will reduce the temptation to check into your life back home and helps you to be more present in the moment.

Practice niksen on a daily basis

On holiday, our brain is inclined to sabotage our downtime, because it's still in work mode. This is why it's so important to train your brain to relax every day. Dutch neurologist and author Dr Erik Scherder says a holiday offers only a temporary solution to work stress. It is more effective to find ways to manage stress in your life with regular breaks. Put an effort into taking time out every day – even on holiday.

Distract your brain

If your mind keeps on firing thoughts, dedicate yourself to an easy physical activity that requires attention but few cognitive skills, such as wandering through a quaint little town, sketching or doodling, or snorkelling.

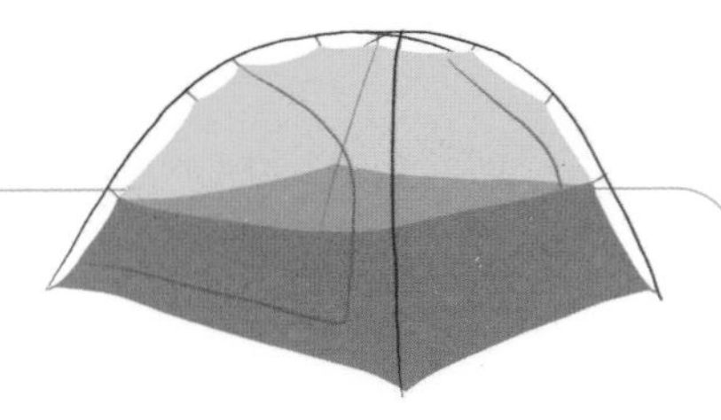

Try Camping

The Dutch are avid campers and, despite its modest size, the Netherlands has over a thousand designated campsites, where people niks the day away. Camping is about going back to basics, without the comfort and luxuries of your home.

There is no space for Netflix, wifi, a dishwasher or games console, but if you're lucky you'll get a sky full of stars, and the fresh smell and beautiful sounds of nature. Your only obligations at camp are sleeping, eating and washing the dishes. There are no appointments or places to go, just huge stretches of time to enjoy nature, to read and to daydream. You can simply be.

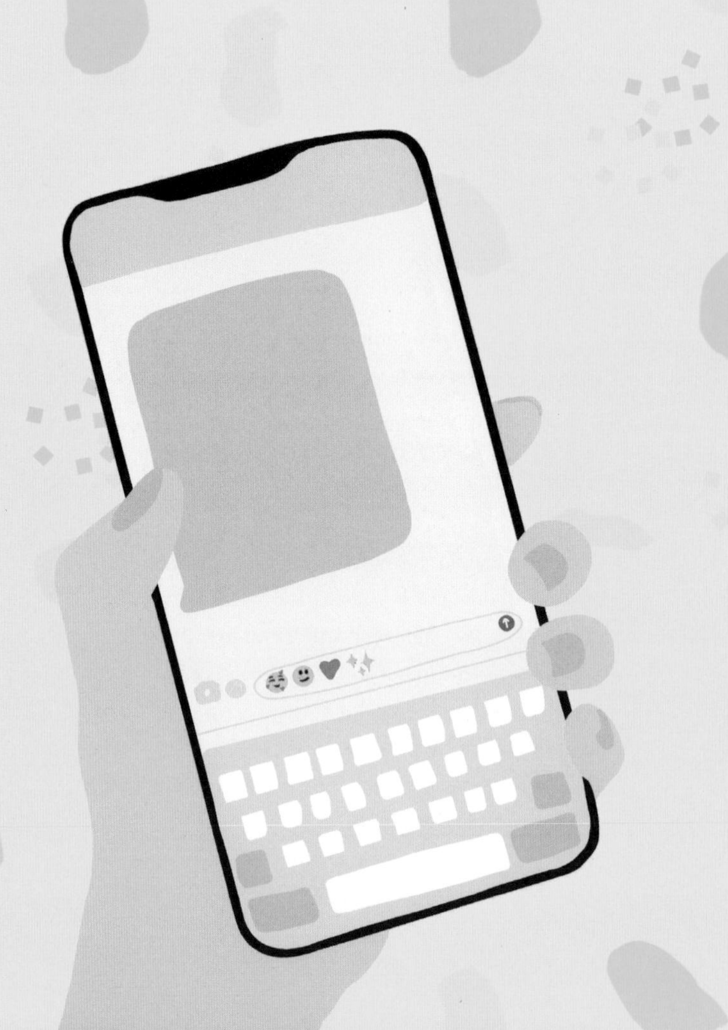

Niksen Online

The average person spends between two and four hours per day on their smartphone, and even though many of us wish we spent less time, we find it difficult to disconnect. How often have you been distracted by the ping of a WhatsApp notification, then ended up browsing through the feeds of your Instagram friends, clicking on an article someone on Facebook shared, or mindlessly scrolling through Twitter?

If we want to spend less time on our phone, we can keep the display in black and white and disable the notifications for social media. But wouldn't it be better to regain control of our attention and enjoy our daily timeouts without feeling the constant urge to check the phone? Take pleasure in being undistracted, uninterrupted and unavailable for a while.

A manageable digital diet

More so than a crash diet, where you fully unplug from your life online, it's important to make small changes that last. By reducing your screen usage and the amount of information flooding your brain, you will create more headspace and time for niksen. Limit messaging to lost moments such as during your commute or when you're waiting for a dentist appointment, and put a cap on your time online.

- Decide which groups are a waste of your time and say your goodbyes. Mute all other groups. Sometimes calling someone can gets things resolved faster and out of your head.

- Remove social media and streaming apps from your phone. You will keep your accounts, but can only access them through the browser.

- Go analogue and try slow reading. Pick up a printed newspaper or magazine, or read a physical book instead of an ebook.

- Use the 'Night Shift' option on your phone to mute notifications and calls in the evening, and make the screen less distracting.

- Declutter your home screen by deleting irrelevant apps or news sources and blogs that are not contributing to your wellbeing.

- Try an app that helps you stay away from your phone while you focus on your work, that helps limit your screen time, or that blocks your internet browser.

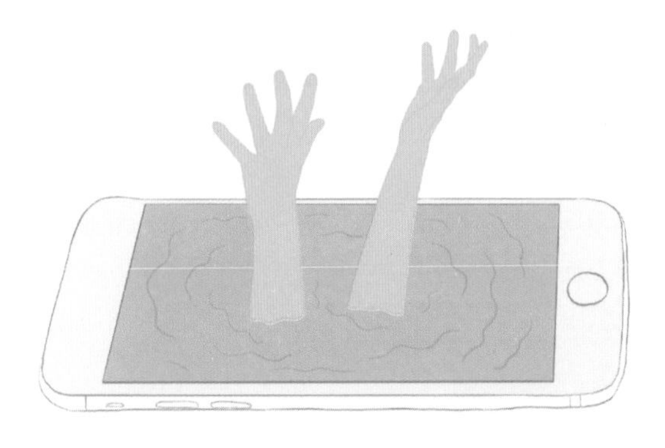

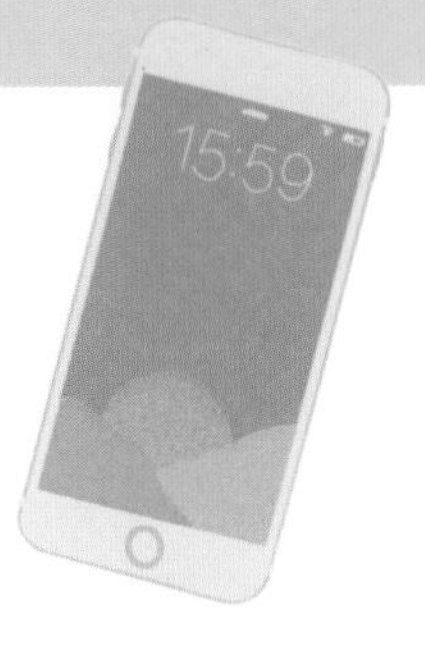

EXERCISE

ATTENTION DEFICIT AND MINDLESS SCROLLING

Every time you check Instagram or another social media platform, keep track of the minutes spent and ask yourself:

'Is this really worth my time?

Does it bring me enough for the time I'm investing in it?

Isn't there something else I would rather spend my time on?'

A simple solution is to allocate a set time to check your social media and respond to messages, rather than scrolling constantly throughout the day.

NIKSEN FOR YOU

Sometimes it feels as though there just aren't enough hours in the day for any me-time. Whether it's a demanding job, your children, a family member, friend, or even a pet, there's always someone else's needs to put above your own. In this chapter we look at ways to make niksen work for everyone.

Niksen for Me, Myself and I

Hanging out with friends can be fun, and can take your mind off worries about work or about life in general. But if you seek a more profound, sensory experience, it is better that you are on your own. It's simply harder to turn inwards if there's another person there. The following tips and exercises can help you find the peace of mind to make your personal downtime count.

How to face feelings of FOMO

Staying in while all your friends are going to a party doesn't mean you have a boring life. It's the FOMO (the fear of missing out) that is messing with your head, even though it was your own decision. You feel restless, obsessively scrolling through social media posts in which your friends look more beautiful and happy than ever before (which they affirm with the hashtag #bestnightever). And there goes your relaxing me-time . . .

Of course, it doesn't *have* to be like that. Stop wasting your energy thinking about what you are missing out on and:

- Remember that you will only get to see the highs, not the lows. The selfies you see may not offer a realistic view of what the event is actually like.

- Accept that you can't join every single get-together. Today you have decided to do something else, and that is to indulge in absolutely nothing.

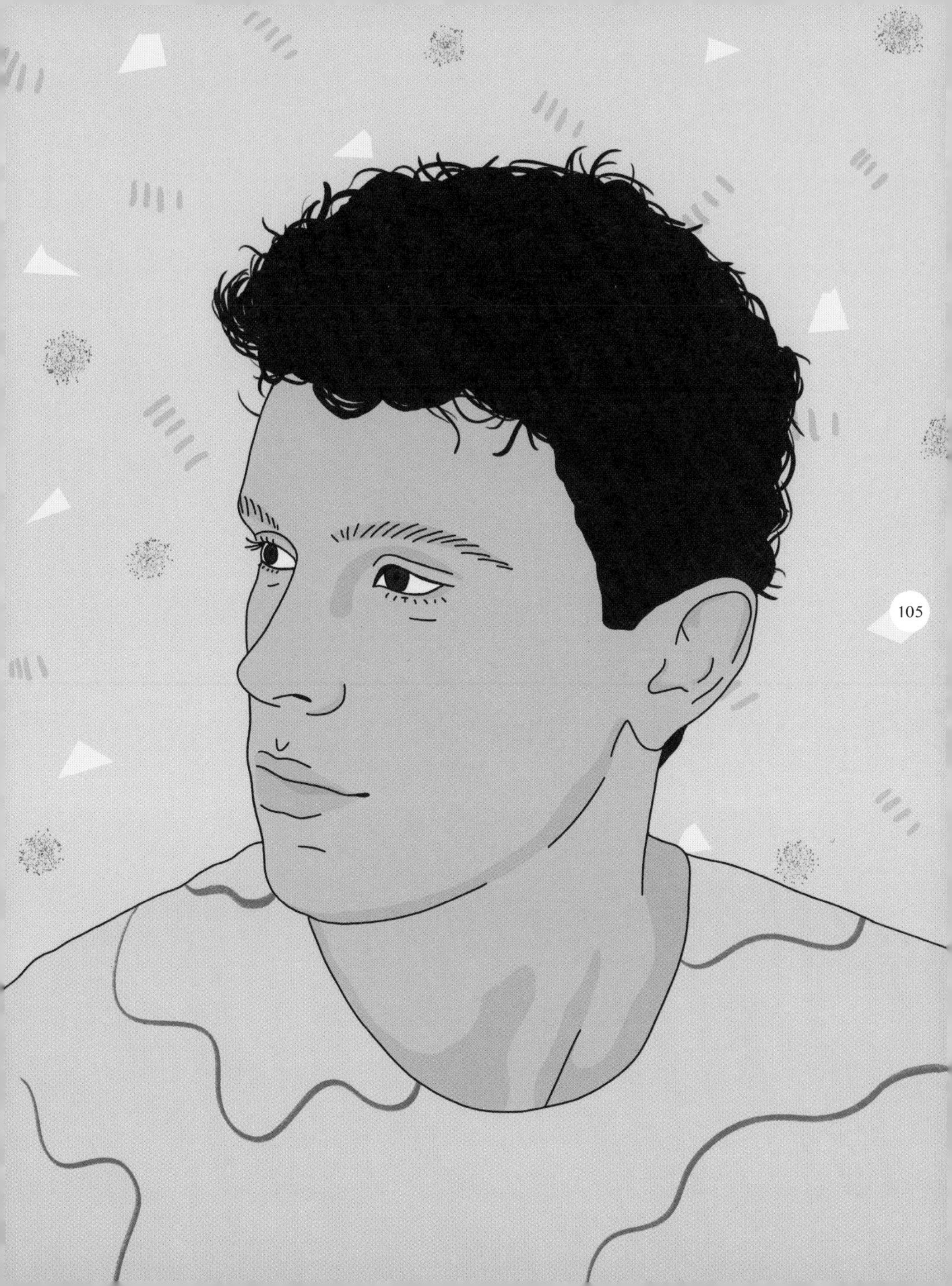

EXERCISE

THE SAFETY BLANKET

You can't afford to join friends for lunch or don't have enough energy to meet someone for the evening, so why not make staying in really count? Next time you settle in to some potentially unsettling alone time, leave your phone in another room or tuck it out of sight in a drawer. Gift yourself one comforting item that requires two hands – perhaps a book or a hot drink. Focus on this item and take care to slow your breathing, encouraging you to unwind. Soon enough, pure JOMO (the joy of missing out) will start kicking in.

As you know, to niks, you first need to clear the mind, and it is much easier to achieve this by pushing away unhelpful distractions and reverting to simple pleasures that wholly occupy us.

In Chapter 7 (see page 122) you will find more activities and exercises that help reduce anxiety and achieve a niksen state of mind.

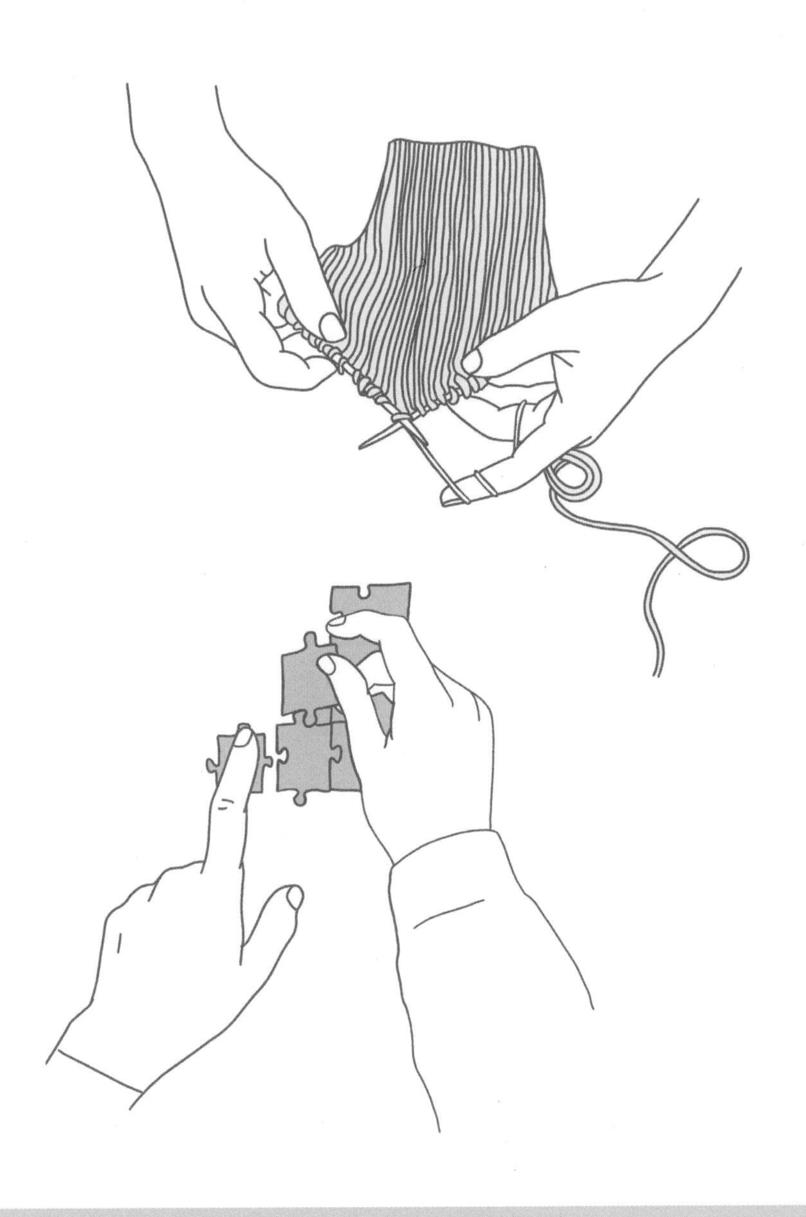

EXERCISE

PEOPLE-WATCHING

People in the Netherlands love to people-watch – *mensen kijken*. In spring, when the sun emerges, the Dutch appear from their houses and flock onto terraces where the seats are ideally lined up in rows, facing the street. It is an enjoyable way to spend some time on your own, whilst not being alone.

Find a seat on a terrace or a bench in your local park and watch the people go by. Your attention may be caught by a beautiful coat, someone's haircut or a facial expression. You know nothing more about these people other than what you can see, but you might start to spin theories about them.

Are they happy or sad, stressed or relaxed, interesting or boring? Don't hold back if your mind starts making up the reasons behind your observations, creating a patchwork of individual stories.

Is it important that your theories are accurate? Not at all. By making up your own stories you stimulate creative thinking.

Should you be discreet? Yes.

Don't follow or stare at people; this exercise is not about them.

EXERCISE

FIND YOUR FLOW

Simple tasks that require little cognitive power and allow for daydreaming may boost your creativity. In her book *The Artist's Way*, Julia Cameron advises readers to commit to weekly 'artist dates'.

An artist date is time spent alone doing something that excites you creatively. Even if this is just a walk outside or a daydream on the sofa, it's important to do it by yourself so that you are influenced only by your own experience.

Spending time on your own is essential in unblocking your creativity, says Cameron, and can help you see things in a different light.

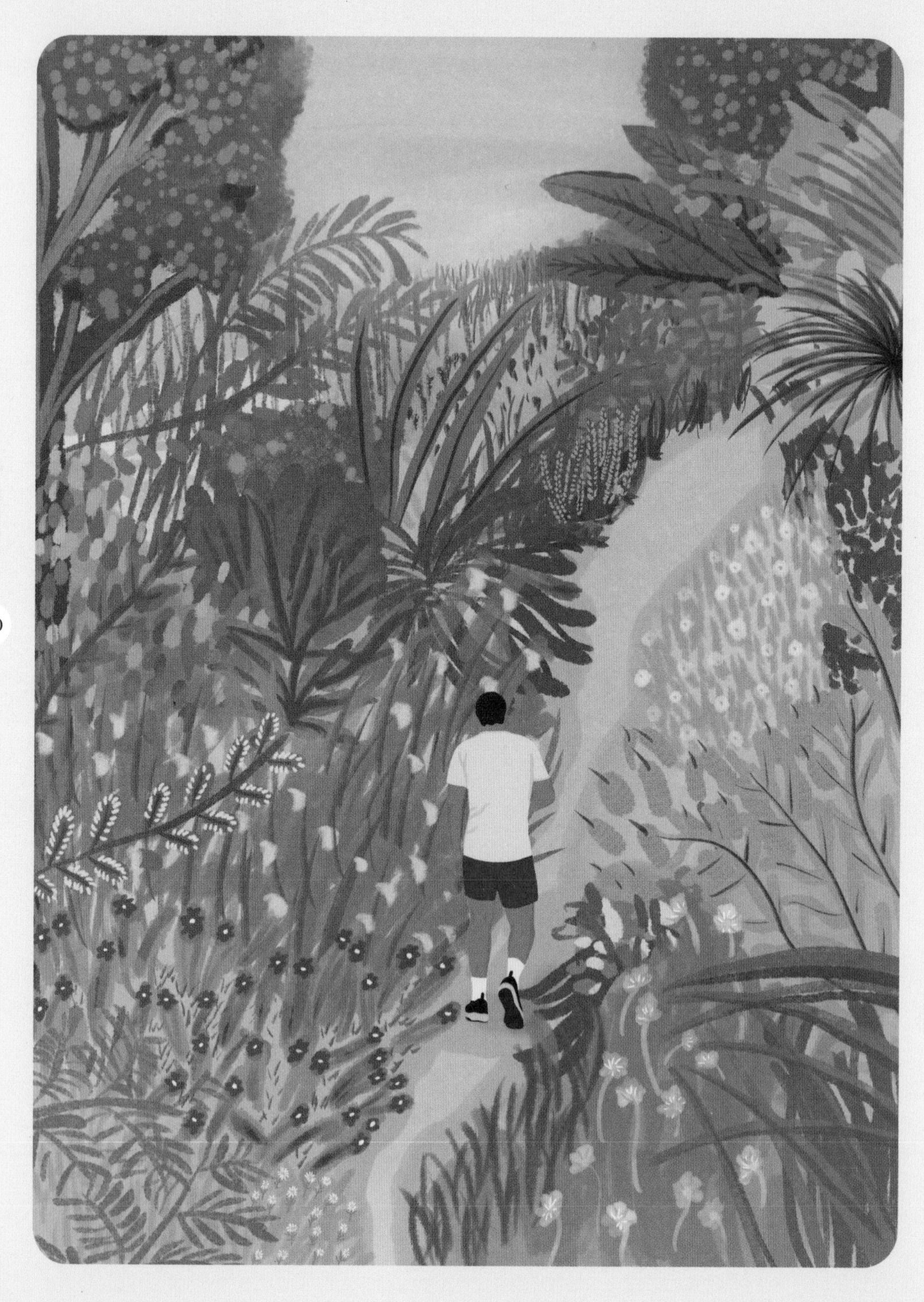

EXERCISE

UITWAAIEN ('HEAD OUT IN THE WIND')

When you feel stressed, angry or depleted of energy, staying inside often won't make you feel any better. You need to get some fresh air, and this is where *uitwaaien* comes in: the act of going out in windy weather as a way to refresh yourself and clear your mind.

Go to the park, a green area or the beach, and face the elements.

Let the wind flush your cheeks, and jump into a puddle if it happens to rain.

It can provide just the reset you need.

Niksen for Parents

It's not always easy to find the right balance between family, work and personal downtime. You want to get your tasks done, but at the same time you want to give your children the attention and time they need, while also taking care of domestic chores and spending time with your partner. In our attempt to manage it all, we sometimes forget that we also need time to relax on our own.

If you feel you are in need of more personal downtime, you may be interested to hear how Dutch parents do it.

Juggling working hours

The Dutch enjoy the shortest working week in the world, with flexible working hours considered a basic right rather than a luxury, especially for parents, who tend to share childcare responsibilities. Many women see working fewer hours as a lifestyle choice rather than a leap backwards in their emancipation, especially when kids enter the picture. And Dutch dads often try to squeeze their working hours into just four days, which allows them to take care of their kids at least one day a week. This day is lovingly called the *Papadag*, meaning 'daddy day'.

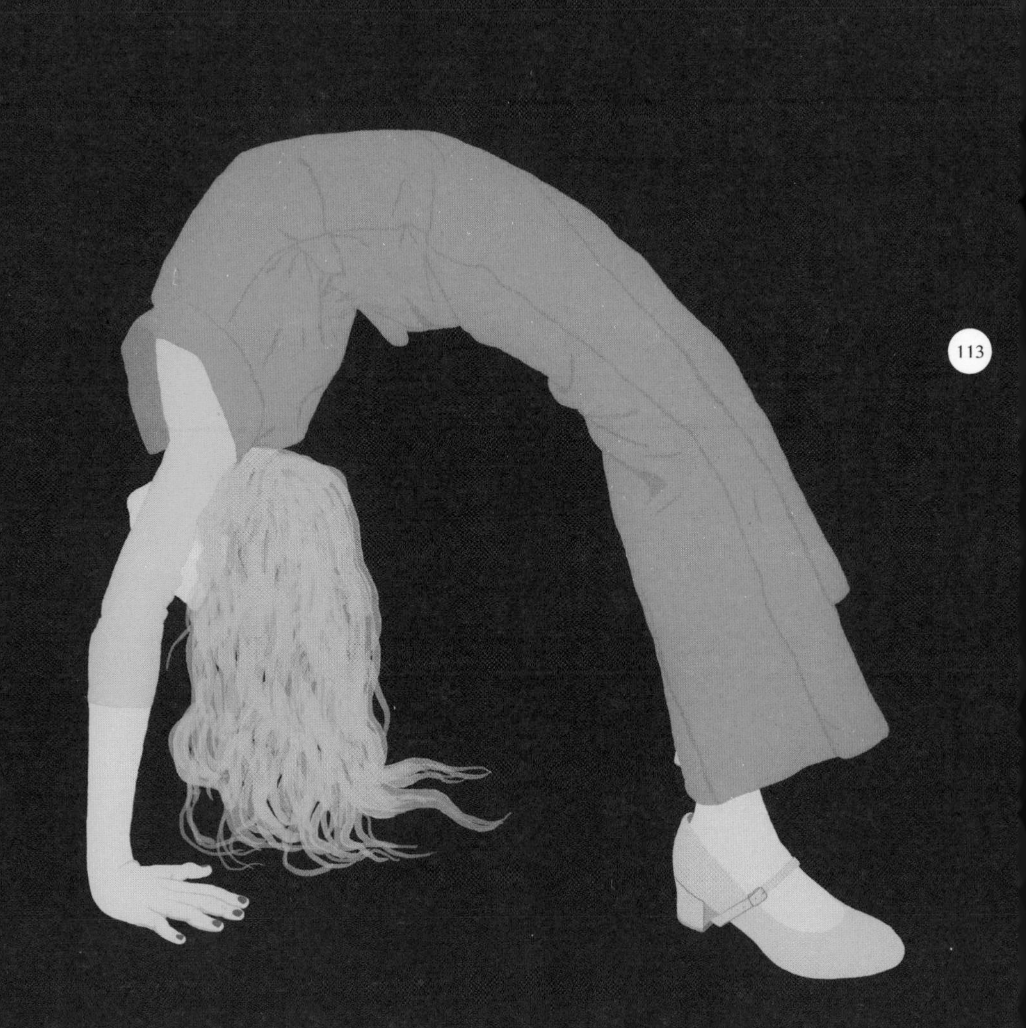

Allowing both mums and dads to spend more time with their kids, as well as pencilling in time for themselves, has had a beneficial impact on family life and is almost certainly a factor in Dutch children scoring amongst the happiest in the world (see page 118).

Discuss with your employer the options for flexible working hours. Can you fit your work into a 4-day week, work from home or even cut working hours? Try to find a way of working that allows you to share parenting duties with your partner.

Be realistic about parenthood

There is an argument that, compared to parents in the US and UK, Dutch parents have a more realistic perspective on parenthood, and are more forgiving of their own shortfalls. Perhaps it's down to their *nuchtere volksaard* – their pragmatic nature – but you won't often hear a Dutch mother expressing guilt about the amount of time she has spent with her children. She will acknowledge that it's important to find time for herself outside motherhood and work, as a happy and relaxed parent allows for a happier child.

Accept that you can't be everywhere at the same time. Sometimes there is a big project at work that needs more attention; sometimes your family requires more focus. All you can do is your best.

Be smart about how you divide your time

- **Cut yourself some slack.** Leave the laundry hanging if there's no time to fold or iron it. Some chores can wait until the weekend.

- **Accept help.** If you can afford it, hire someone to babysit the kids or to help with chores in and around the house. And if the grandparents offer help, take it! This will allow you to spend some time with your partner or by yourself.

- **Collaborate.** Work with your partner to create simple routines that will save you both time and headspace. For example, on weekdays they will watch the kids while you prepare dinner.

- **Protect your boundaries.** If you don't have time to make costumes for the Christmas play or bake cookies for the summer fair, be honest.

- **Make your work commute me-time.** Listen to an audiobook, podcast or your favourite music on repeat. Is the office close enough to walk? Then leave early and take it easy to really enjoy this moment of me-time.

- **Get up before your kids do.** Allow yourself 20 minutes of alone time, to quietly enjoy your coffee, read the newspaper and prepare for the day.

- **Make time for nothing.** One evening a week, ask your partner to take the kids out so you have the house to yourself. Claim the sofa, take a bath or fall asleep – do whatever you want that is not a chore or obligation; this is your night.

Niksen for Kids

Surveys by the World Health Organisation (2010), UNICEF (2007, 2013) and the OECD (2015) have consistently highlighted the perks of a childhood in the Netherlands. In a more recent HBSC study (2020), Dutch 15-year olds reported an open and supportive relationship with their mum (90 per cent) and dad (81 per cent), as opposed to an overall average of 80 and 65 per cent respectively. They also tend to experience fewer mental health problems, less problematic use of social media and less bullying. So why are Dutch kids such a content bunch? There are indications that in the Netherlands niksen is as important for kids as it is for adults.

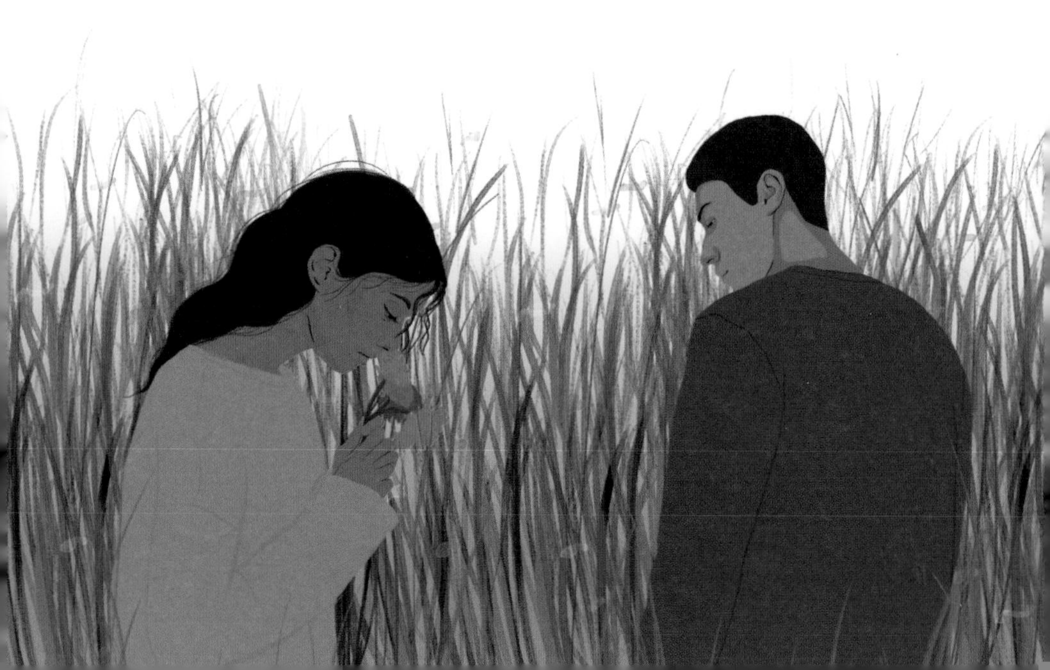

Thank God it's Monday

It is common in the UK and US for children to spend their weekends doing homework and being driven between football training, swimming lessons, a piano recital and of course their weekly Japanese class. Because you want to give your child the best start in life, don't you?

Most Dutch parents adhere to a more laid-back style of parenting. Dutch kids are encouraged to play outside; they cycle to school unsupervised, rain or shine; and there is less pressure to take part in numerous scheduled activities. In fact, *betutteling* (cosseting) – where kids are treated as vulnerable creatures who can't think for themselves and need to be monitored every single minute – is disapproved of. Basically, Dutch parents incorporate a great deal more niksen moments into their children's lives.

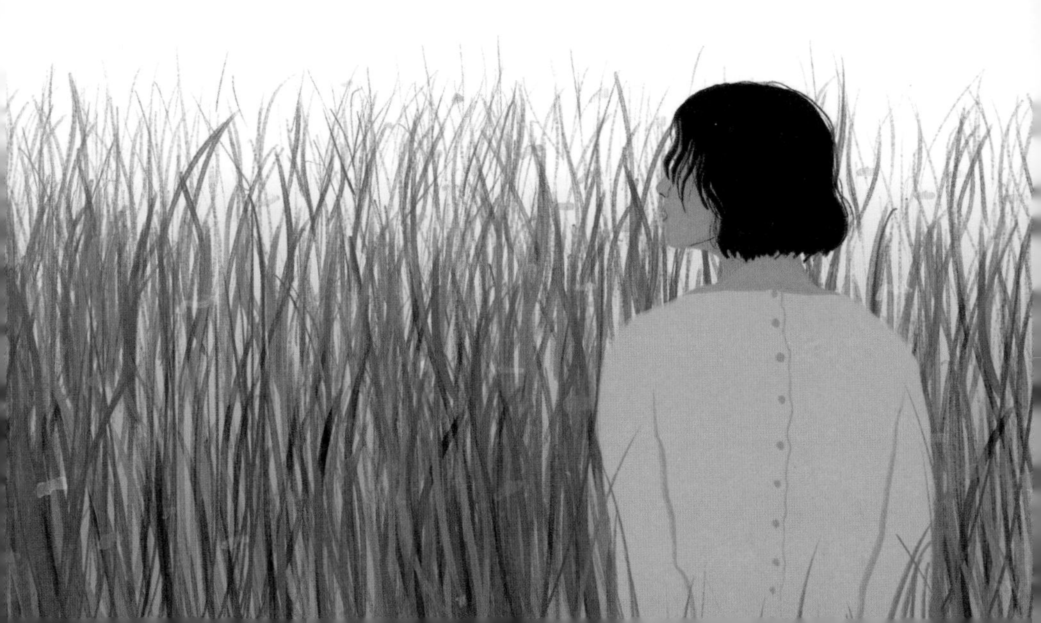

Be less concerned about your kid being the smartest

You might question whether such an upbringing promotes professional success later in life. Like all parents, the Dutch have great ambitions for their children. But happiness and the development of social skills are still considered more important than the cultivation of talent or academic excellence.

Many Dutch people believe a happy and playful child is more likely to grow into an independent, social and eventually successful human being. Kids are not pressured into taking up a particular hobby or skill that their parents consider 'useful'. If they want to play football with their friends instead of taking piano lessons, that's fine. Dutch children also have less homework (and thus more free time) than their peers in the US and UK.[1] If you feel urged to educate or entertain your child all the time, then remember it is particularly in those moments of boredom that children are triggered to be more creative and enjoy themselves.

And it's hard to argue with the numbers: in an extensive survey by the Centraal Bureau voor de Statistiek (CBS) in 2015, 94 per cent of 12–18 year olds in the Netherlands reported feeling content and happy with their lives; and an OECD report from 2018 showed that over 93 per cent of 11–15 years old scored above average life satisfaction.

---

1 *According to the 'Health and Behaviour in School-aged Children' study (HBSC/WHO, 2010), Dutch children experience relatively little pressure (5%) from school, compared to children in the UK (15%) and USA (18%).*

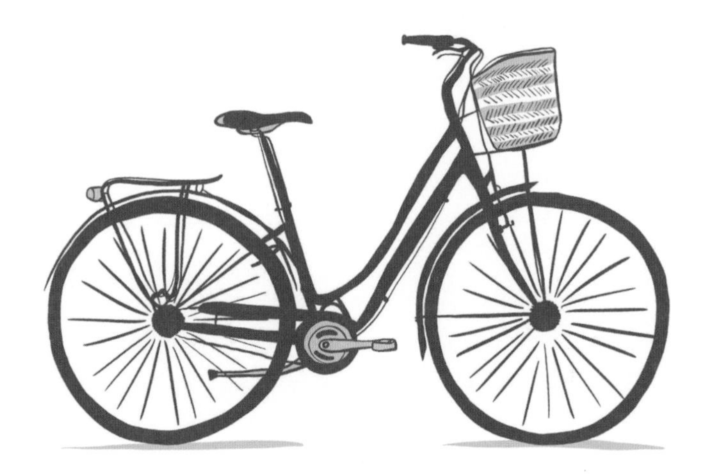

Role-modelling

Drop one or two things from your own schedule to set a good example to your child. If you tell them it's important to rest and relax, don't demonstrate the opposite by running around like a headless chicken. Role model for your kids how to take care of yourself, by taking time out. Discuss with your child what they enjoy doing most, and see if you can cancel or postpone a few of the activities they take less pleasure in. Spend these hours on a meaningful activity, just for the two of you, such as reading a story or taking a walk. There's nothing wrong with teaching kids how to entertain themselves; even in boredom they can learn a lot.

The importance of rest

Research shows that Dutch babies sleep a lot. And in 2015, a study published in the *European Journal of Developmental Psychology* found that, in comparison to their peers in the US, Dutch infants are more likely to be happy and easier to soothe, while in the latter half of their first year, US infants are typically more active and vocal. The researchers believe these results reflect the parents' different and unique cultural values. Parents in the US emphasise the importance of stimulation, exposing their kids to a wide variety of new experiences to promote independence. Dutch parents, on the other hand, are more likely to incorporate children into activities at home, attaching more importance to rest, regularity and niksen.

EXERCISE

BRUSH YOUR TEETH TOGETHER

An ideal self-care exercise that is also a shared experience, teeth-brushing will help both you and your brushing buddy find a peaceful moment to be together in harmony.

This is something that's already part of everyone's daily routine, and a therapeutic ritual that perfectly readies us all for bed.

A NIKS STATE OF MIND

Congratulations! You're well on your way to a happy, niksen-filled life. You've learned how to set priorities, carve out more free time in your schedule, and be smarter about managing your own moments of niksen. In this final chapter, we look at how to successfully build up and sustain the practice of doing nothing.

How to Do Nothing

You have scheduled time and given yourself permission to do nothing, but the act itself may feel awkward at first. Counterintuitive even, if you're used to doing something all the time. Start with a few minutes, push through the discomfort, and work up to an hour or more a day. Try the following exercises to help you cross the threshold.

Active relaxation exercises

If you are restless and constantly dragged along by your raging thoughts, you can distract your mind by adding some movement to your relaxation ritual. This can be an easy walk around town, a form of 'moving meditation' such as yoga or tai chi, or a muscle relaxation exercise (see page 69).

Passive relaxation exercises

Keep your body in relaxation mode and focus on what you can hear, feel, see and smell. Our senses are great tools with which to get deeper into relaxation. You could also do a body scan (see overleaf), have a massage, listen to classical music, do a visualisation exercise (see page 55), or watch the moving leaves of a tree or the clouds roll by as you let your mind meander.

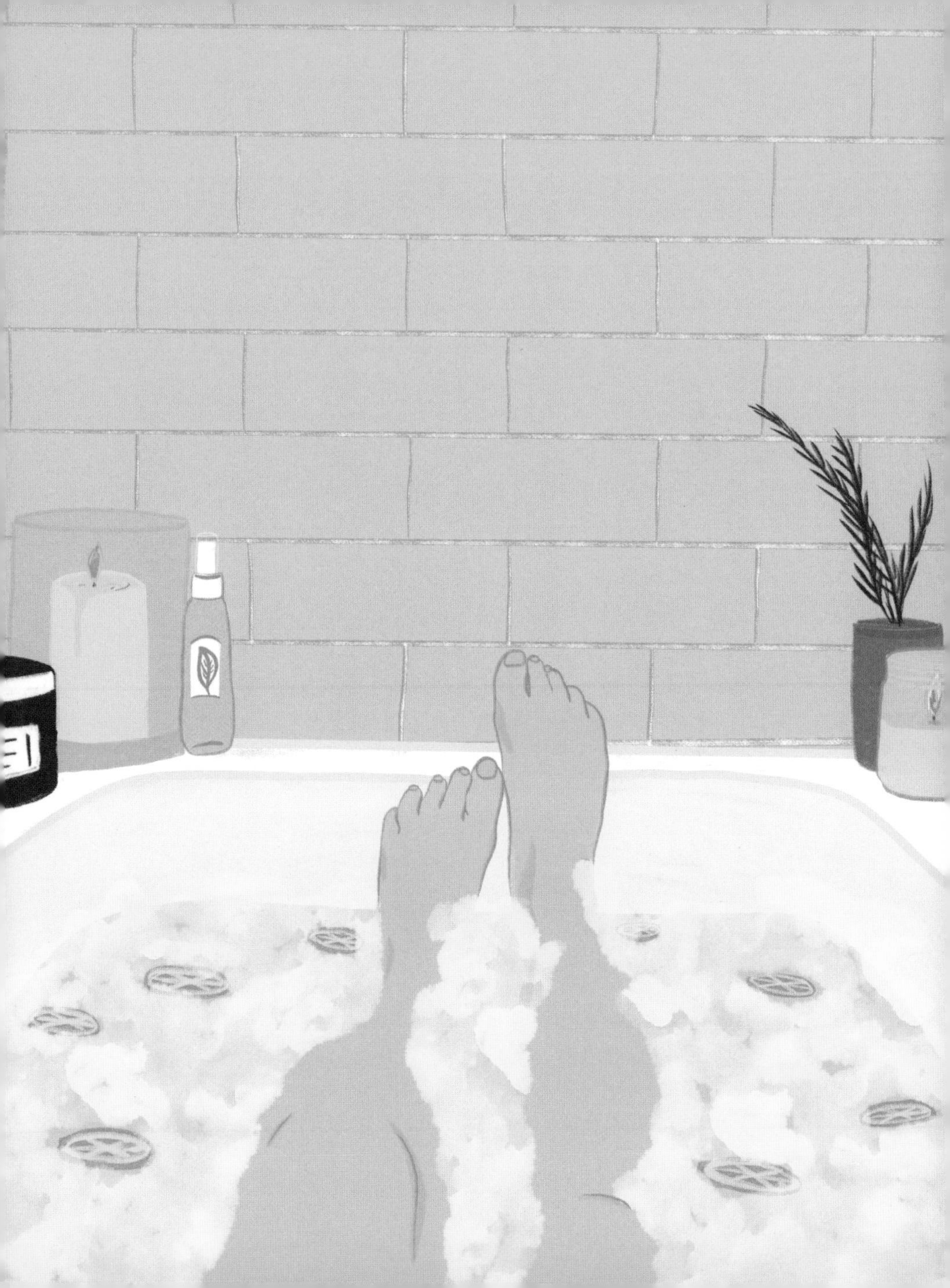

EXERCISE

SENSORY BODY SCAN

This is a classic relaxation exercise that can help you arrive in a niksen state of mind after a busy day, and allows you to process the messages your body is trying to send to you. Use the body scan as a bridge between your daily commitments and personal downtime. With a relaxed feeling and a quietened mind, it becomes much easier to sink into moments of niksen.

You can do this scan while walking if you want to make it active, but below we'll focus on doing it while lying down.

STEP ① Find a quiet spot outside. The sounds, scents and feel of your surroundings will help you stay awake: the breeze that caresses your face, the smell of fresh-mown grass.

STEP ② Place your hands on your belly and focus on your breathing. Visualise the fresh air entering your body.

STEP ③ Once your breathing is calm and relaxed, start directing your attention downwards, to your feet. Don't move, but take a moment to connect.

STEP ④ Every time you get distracted by a sound, scent, feeling or thought, try not to linger on it, but gently bring your attention back to your body.

STEP ⑤ Slowly move your focus upwards to your ankles, calves, knees, and so on, all the way up to your face.

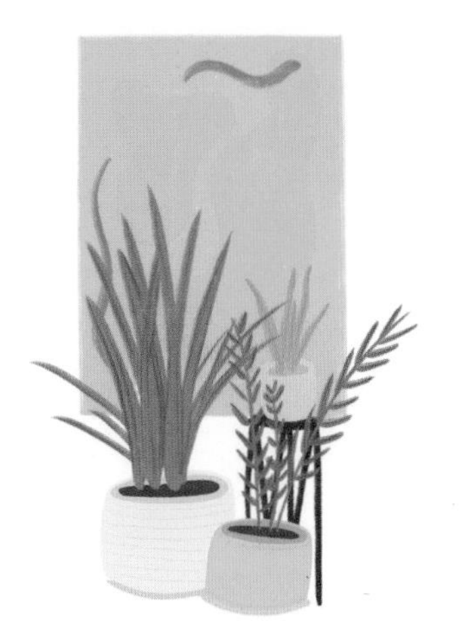

Seek beauty

To arrive in a state of deep relaxation that triggers creativity, you want to encourage your mind to wander in a way that's inspiring and imaginative. Surround yourself with beautiful art, play music or go out into nature to soothe your heart and awaken your senses.

When I'm at home alone, I love to lay down on the sofa and watch my *Birds*. I bought the painting several years ago, from Japanese artist Hidenori Mitsue, who took his inspiration from *The Goldfinch* by old Dutch master Carel Fabritius – and it never ceases to surprise me. As time passes by, I watch how the light falling in through the high windows continually changes its colours and shadows, and at times creates the illusion that my birds will take off, escaping the canvas and flying out the window.

If you're trapped in an uninspiring office building and need a plan B, you may resort to your imagination and find beauty in a daydream or recall your happy place in your mind's eye.

EXERCISE

CHASING CLOUDS

People in the Netherlands pride themselves on their beautiful cloud-filled skies, which have been captured on the canvases of numerous great artists, from Brueghel and Rembrandt to Vermeer and Van Gogh. I wonder if this obsession is not just a way to ignore the fact that the Dutch landscape is rather plain, but it is true that watching the clouds roll by makes for an ideal niksen activity.

Bring a blanket and a pot of tea, lay flat on your back and see what stories you can associate with the whimsical forms that move past like a film.

Meditative making

If you don't feel drawn to meditation, but do want to experience a meditative state of mind and the associated benefits of reduced anxiety and stress, consider taking up knitting or quilting. They may sound boring, but don't rule them out just yet. Because of their rhythmic and repetitive nature, these almost automatic crafts can help you achieve a state of 'flow', which has been proven to boost mood and reduce anxiety. Finding a single focus is a helpful first step to letting your mind roam.

Flow was first described by psychologist Mihály Csíkszentmihályi as 'a state of concentration and complete absorption with the activity at hand and the situation'. You are so involved in the activity that nothing else seems to matter, and you will feel relaxed, comforted and contemplative.

Similar effects can be obtained from drawing or taking a walk. Commit to doing it frequently (at least three times a week) and use it as a stepping stone to a calmer mind, which is sufficiently at ease to do nothing.

Stop multitasking

Whatever you choose to do, give it your full attention. Don't pick up the phone if you are writing in your journal; don't tidy up while you are trying to relax and listen to music. Multitasking requires a lot of energy and headspace, and it is known to make us even more restless. Doing one thing at a time relieves your brain and makes for a more genuinely productive day.

Practice mindfulness for an undisturbed mind

Meditation and mindfulness exercises can help you gain more control over your mind and maximise the effects of niksen. Meditate in a group or listen to a guided meditation to ease your practice and get deeper into the relaxation, or keep it simple with an observation exercise such as the one opposite.

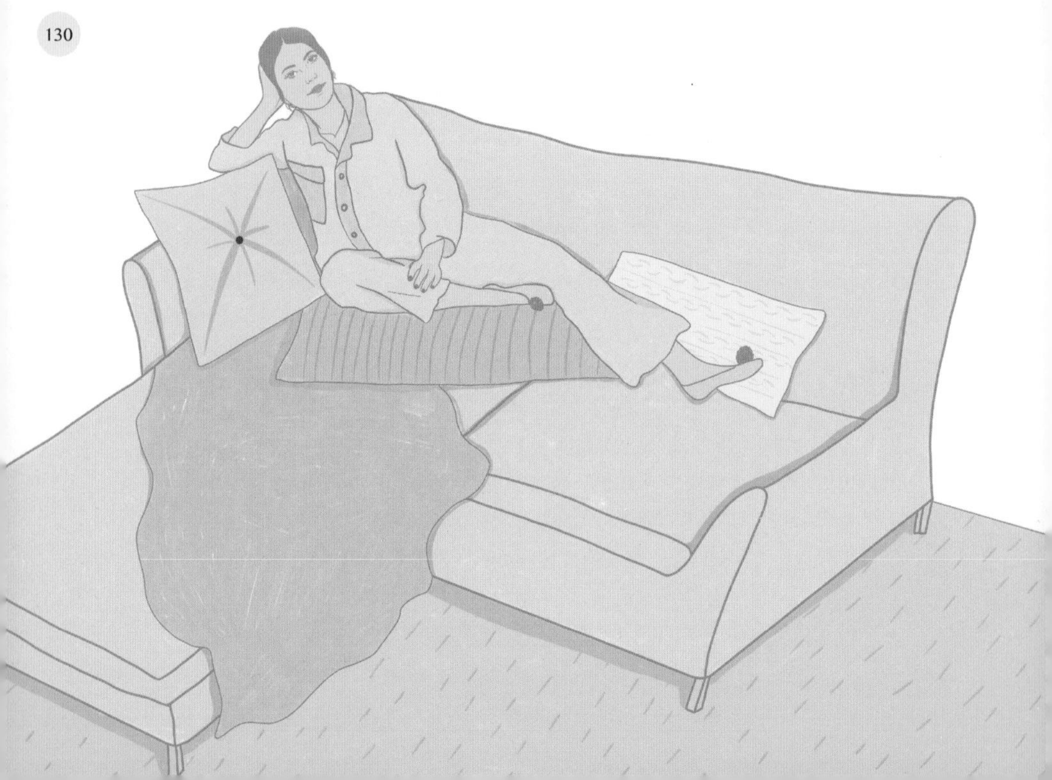

EXERCISE

RAINDROPS ON YOUR WINDOW

Make the best of a grey and rainy day by watching how the raindrops travel down the windowpane.

Sit and watch how the droplets land on the glass, then roll down, meet one another, coalesce and continue their way to the bottom of the pane. You can do this exercise at home, in the car or on the bus, passing time by following the raindrops' paths.

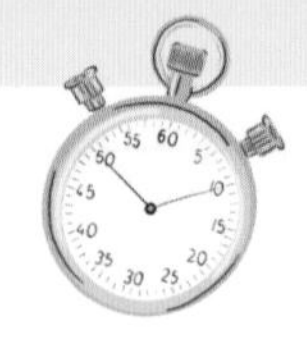

EXERCISE

THE TWO-MINUTE RULE

I love this simple yet effective trick by by productivity guru and author of *Getting Things Done* David Allen. When a new task comes in and you can do it in less than two minutes, focus on doing it right away. Don't leave it lingering in the back of your mind, claiming headspace. Give it all of your attention and feel that sense of achievement from getting it done and dusted.

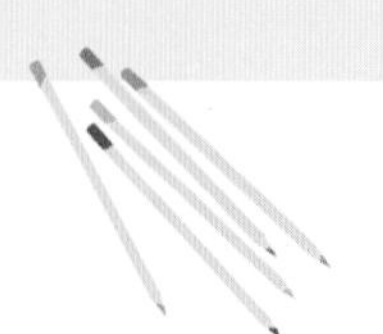

EXERCISE

STAY INSPIRED

Do you feel that there is a part of you that has been lost? What did you love doing as a child that you no longer do? This could be drawing, reading, writing or singing. Choose anything that makes you feel like time does not exist and note this down.

For example: I find happiness in a daydream, in reading poetry, in how my mind comes up with the most creative thoughts when I try to put them on paper. Keep these notes nearby, at your desk or pinned onto the fridge, as subtle reminders on how to stay inspired.

The Importance of Self-care

Taking time out every day is one way to take care of yourself. But to cope with stress you should also make sure you get enough sleep, eat healthily, exercise regularly and reduce the number of commitments you undertake. We all know this, but many don't live up to it. When everyone seems to want something from us, it's hard to put our own interests first.

Our body and mind are connected. If you've had a rough night, if you're hungry or ill, you'll be more susceptible to stress and negative feelings. Decide what you could cancel this week. How can you get out of your head and into your body? Who can you ask for help? How can you carve out more time for nothing? And how can you improve your sleep?

Early bird catches the worm

A 2016 study by the University of Michigan showed that Dutch people sleep longer than anyone else in the world. The researchers believe their sleep quality is derived from the fact that the Dutch have dinner early, usually no later than 6pm, which allows their body to digest their evening meal. The study also showed a direct correlation between an early bedtime and a quality night's sleep: the later a person stays up, the less quality sleep they get.

Try to create a bedtime routine by going to bed no later than 11pm and minimising your screen time after 8pm. Try to bring forward your evening meal and eat a light snack before bedtime. If you wake early, don't go back to sleep as you'll feel worse when the alarm goes off. Instead, use those extra minutes to gently awaken your body and mentally prepare for the day.

A Good Night's Sleep

Country	Average night's sleep
Netherlands	8 hr 05 min
Australia	8 hr 01 min
Canada	7 hr 58 min
UK	7 hr 53 min
USA / Spain	7 hr 50 min
Germany	7 hr 41 min
Japan	7 hr 30 min
Singapore	7 hr 23 min

Source: Walch, Olivia J., Cochran, Amy and Forger, Daniel B., 'A Global Quantification of 'Normal' Sleep Schedules Using Smartphone Data', Science Advances, *May 2016.*[1]

---

1 *The window between the longest and shortest night's sleep is not huge, but the researchers say every half an hour of sleep makes a big difference in terms of cognitive function and long-term health.*

EXERCISE

SUPPORTIVE TOUCH

Just as a baby calms down when being cuddled in its mother's arms, our own body also responds to the physical gesture of warmth and care. If you are going through a rough time, be extra kind to yourself by giving yourself physical support. This causes our brain to release oxytocin and activates our parasympathetic nervous system, which helps to calm us down and provides a sense of security.

①
Lie down somewhere comfortable.

②
Warm your hands by rubbing them together and take three slow, deep breaths.

③
When you're ready, place one hand over your heart, feeling its gentle pressure and warmth. Place your other hand next to it, noticing the difference between one and two hands.

④
Feel the natural rising and falling of your chest as you breathe in and out.

⑤
Make small, soothing circles with your hands.

⑥
Take your time and spend as long on the exercise as you need.

EXERCISE

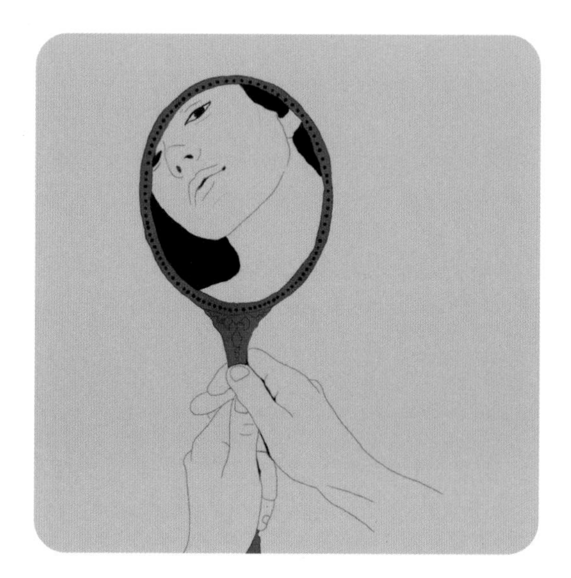

MAKE UP A RITUAL

A ritual helps to make an experience more precious, spiritual and meaningful. If it is performed regularly and feels like an essential comfort or release, a ritual can transform something relatively normal into a special event that you treasure. Brushing your teeth (see page 121), washing your hair, your morning coffee and your Sunday lie-in can all be rituals. Think about something simple (and inexpensive) that you can celebrate easily and consistently, and make it a time for you.

Your Daily Niks Fix

Every day, do at least one of the niksen activities below. If you believe you're too busy for this, reread Chapter 2 (see page 28).

- Lay down, close your eyes and wander off to your happy place (see page 69).
- Take a seat next to the window and watch the clouds go by (see page 128) or the rain fall (see page 131).
- Sit down on a terrace in a lively street and watch the people go by (see page 108).
- Let your breathing calm you (see page 55).
- Look for the beauty in your favourite piece of music or painting (see page 127).
- Spend time in your niksen room (see page 83).
- Get lost in a daydream (see page 109).
- Get outside and enjoy some fresh air (see page 111).
- Eat your lunch in the park (see page 88).

Niksen quickstarters

If you find it difficult to do nothing because you have a lot on your mind or because you haven't been able to fully relax into it yet, find a solo activity that takes your mind off your everyday worries but doesn't require any effort. These gentle pastimes can help you get used to taking time out from the rat race, relaxing and preparing you for the next step: doing absolutely nothing.

- Choose an easy yoga sequence (for example the Five Tibetan Rites or Sun Salutation) and repeat for at least ten minutes.
- Cook a simple recipe you know by heart.
- Run or sprint in short bursts in an empty field or lane.
- Write or draw in your journal.
- Try your luck with knitting.
- Go out for a map-free walk.

None of these activities include a smartphone or computer. Leave your devices at home or place them in flight mode so you're not disturbed by calls or notifications.

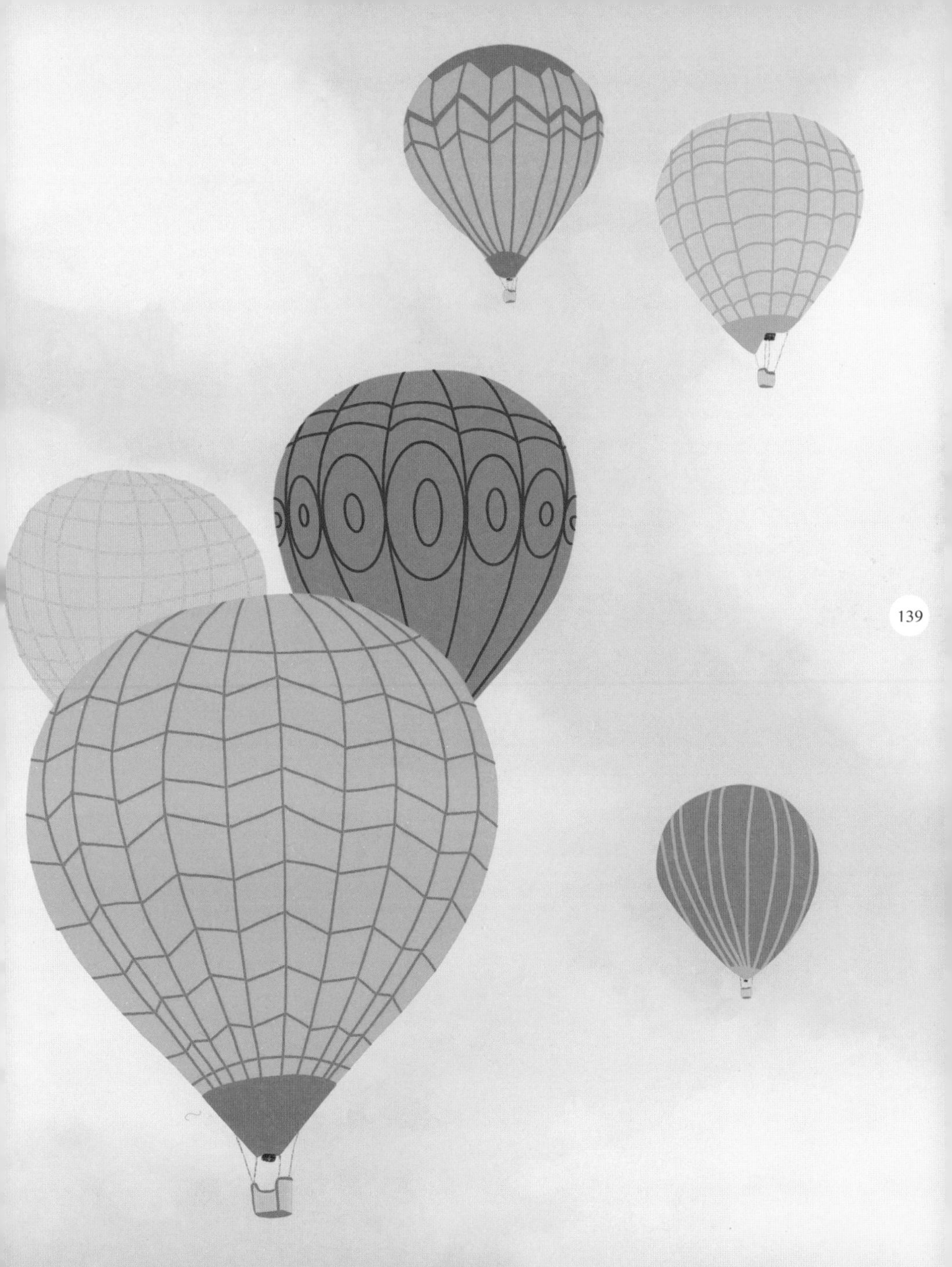

CONCLUSION

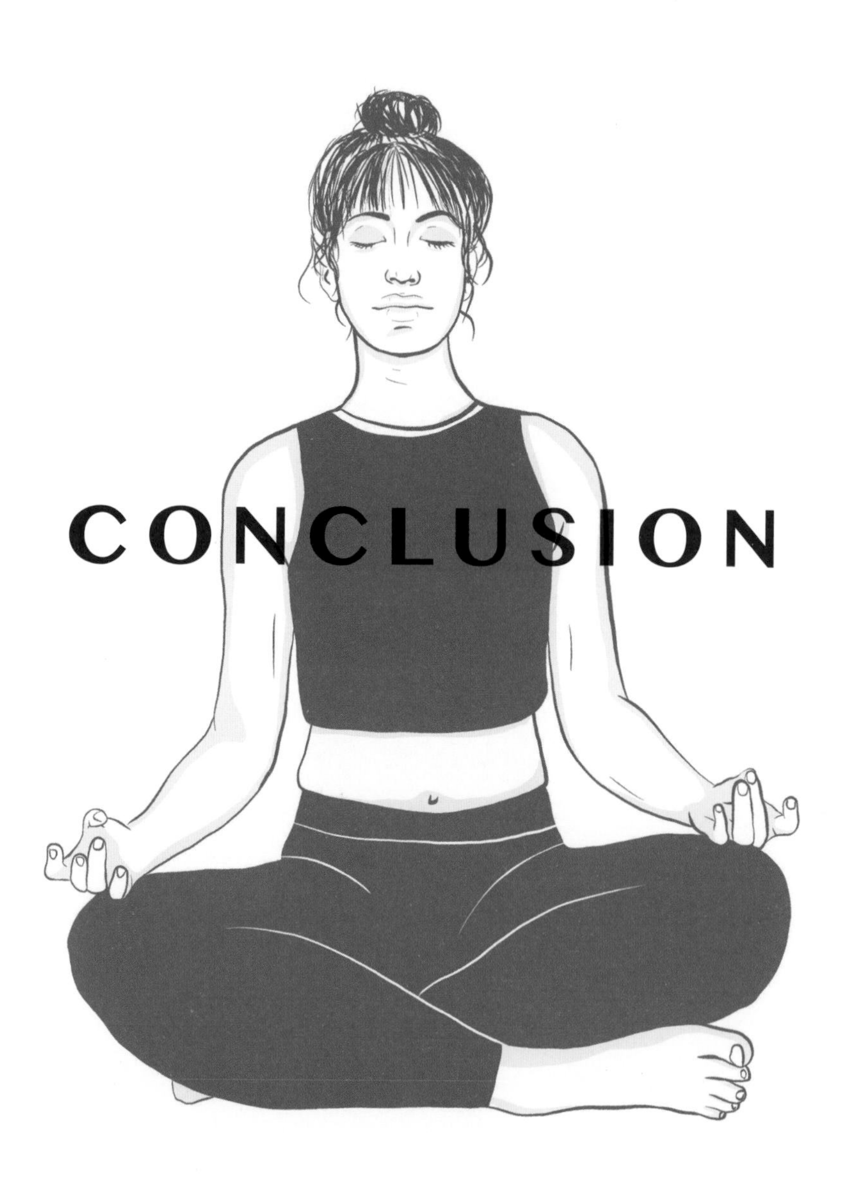

It took me nearly 38 years to realise that being idle is not something to feel guilty or anxious about. To discover the freedom of doing nothing and letting my mind wander without thinking I should be spending my time on 'more useful' things instead.

Don't get me wrong. I'm still juggling commitments between being a diligent worker, a caring mother and a good friend, and sometimes life gets in the way of my personal downtime. I sacrifice quite a few evenings and weekends to work, and there are still days I'm shocked by my screen time.

Just like everyone else I seek a balance between time spent on work, family and relaxation, hoping to minimise stress and frustration. Embracing niksen as a positive practice has helped me to find and sustain this balance. It has changed my priorities and shifted my perception of time. I am more selective in how I organise my days, which surprisingly hasn't increased my procrastination levels, but motivates me to use my work hours more efficiently and effectively – leaving me more downtime to spend as I like.

I hope you feel inspired to embrace your own moments of nothingness. Whenever you sense your free time is being taken away from you, reclaim it gently: prioritise yourself, have the courage to say no, make space by using the techniques described in this book, and indulge in nothingness. To master the art of niksen is to experience the power of pause.

FURTHER RESOURCES

INTERESTING READS

Acosta, Rina Mae and Hutchison, Michele, *The Happiest Kids in the World: Bringing up Children the Dutch Way*, Transworld Publishers, 2017.

Crabbe, Tony, *Busy: How to Thrive in a World of Too Much*, Piatkus, 2014.

Knight, Sarah, *The Life-Changing Magic of Not Giving a F**k*, Quercus Editions, 2015.

Onstad, Katrina, *The Weekend Effect: The Life-Changing Benefits of Taking Time Off and Challenging the Cult of Overwork*, HarperCollins Publishers, 2017.

Sunim, Haemin, *The Things You Can Only See When You Slow Down: How to be Calm in a Busy World*, Penguin, 2018.

HELPFUL APPLICATIONS

Calm: A mindfulness app with guided meditations, nature sounds and sleep stories to help you relax on a busy day and sleep better.

Forest: A productivity app that helps you stay focused and present in blocks of 25 minutes or more. Plant a virtual tree while you focus on your work, or on niksen. Leaving the app halfway through will cause your tree to die.

Stayfocusd: If surfing the web is what's keeping you from completing your tasks, use this URL blocker (in Google Chrome).

Strict Workflow: Based on the Pomodoro Technique (see page 90), this plugin (in Google Chrome) helps you to keep focused on work. Whenever it's time for a break the screen will freeze.

ABOUT THE AUTHOR

Annette Lavrijsen is the former editor of *Women's Health* (Netherlands), and as a freelance journalist she writes mostly on health, psychology and nature. She is also the author of the book *Shinrin-Yoku* (2018), on the Japanese art of forest bathing and the refreshing power of natural mindfulness, which has been translated into five languages. She regularly disconnects from her phone, wifi and daily concerns, in search of new insights and fresh energy and vigour. Annette divides her time between Amsterdam and Barcelona.

THANKS

Writing this book has been a genuine team effort. Thanks to everyone at White Lion Publishing who helped bring Niksen into the world. Special thanks to commissioning editor Zara Anvari, for your trust and patience, to editor Laura Bulbeck, for your helpful edits and for making the writing process flow smoothly as a river, and to Isabel Eeles, for the crisp and clean design. And last but not least, thanks to Brittney Klein and Alissa Levy, your beautiful illustrations have been the icing on the cake.

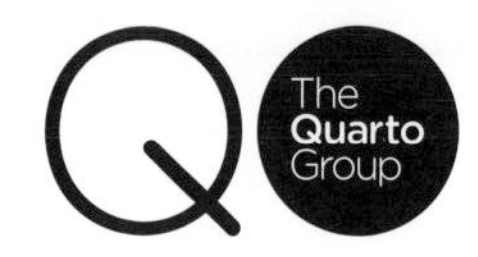

First published in 2020 by White Lion Publishing,
an imprint of The Quarto Group.
The Old Brewery, 6 Blundell Street
London, N7 9BH,
United Kingdom
T (0)20 7700 6700
www.QuartoKnows.com

A catalogue record for this book is available from the British Library.

ISBN 978-0-7112-5523-4
Ebook ISBN 978-0-7112-5524-1

10 9 8 7 6 5 4 3 2 1

Design by Isabel Eeles
Typeset in Lato and Lao MN

Printed in China